Zen and the Art of Medicine

By Dr Victor Denis Purcell

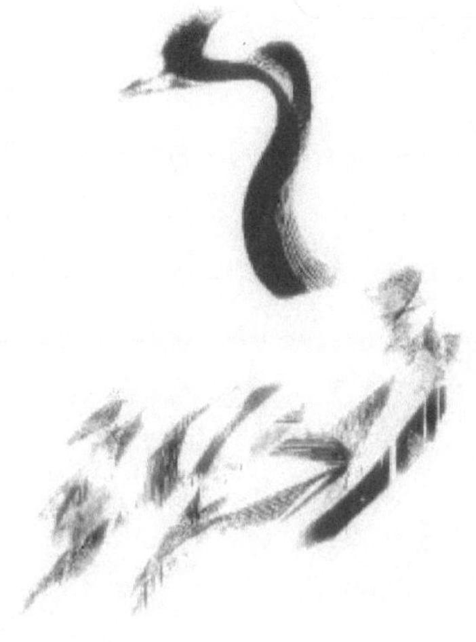

Zen and the Art of Medicine

Dr Víctor Denis Purcell

Published by Dr Víctor Denis Purcell, 2023.

ZEN AND THE ART OF MEDICINE

First edition. October 28, 2023.

Copyright © 2023 Dr Víctor Denis Purcell.

ISBN: 979-8223250913

Written by Dr Víctor Denis Purcell.

Alexander

Introduction:

Amid the ceaseless march of science and progress, the essence of what it means to be human often gets overlooked. However, in the vast expanse of medicine and healing, there lies an intersection where time-honored wisdom meets the advancements of today. At this crossroad, Zen stands as a sentinel, reminding us of the invaluable significance of presence, awareness, and connection.

The role of the healthcare professional is both a privilege and a challenge. Every day, they stand at the interface of life and death, hope and despair. In this role, their spirit bears the collective weight of humanity's most profound moments. But while the responsibility is immense, so too is the risk of burnout and emotional exhaustion. Here, Zen is not merely a palliative but a transformative force. By anchoring oneself in its teachings, professionals can reconnect with their innermost purpose, finding equilibrium amidst the chaos.

Zen, while ancient, is neither arcane nor irrelevant. Instead, it offers practical and profound insights into the modern world. Its meditation practices, honed over millennia, have been shown to alleviate symptoms of depression and anxiety, sharpen cognitive faculties, and even bolster physical well-being. Beyond the empiricism of scientific studies, Zen, at its core, fosters a deeper understanding of oneself and the world.

In light of Zen's teachings, the concept of preventive care acquires a renewed and enriched significance. By emphasizing the intrinsic link between mind and body, Zen advocates for a life of balance, where well-being and purpose coalesce. Rather than waiting for maladies to manifest and then reactively addressing them, the Zen-inspired approach seeks harmony from the outset, foreseeing potential imbalances and remedying them preemptively.

This nuanced perspective on health transcends mere symptom management. Zen invites us to perceive health not as the absence of disease but as the presence of holistic harmony. It's a journey, an ongoing dialogue between patient and healer. As Zen principles permeate modern medicine, they rekindle the core ethos of healthcare – that of mutual respect, deep understanding, and shared purpose.

Yet, such integration isn't without challenges. It demands more than mere knowledge; it requires wisdom. The meticulous rigor of medical science, when paired with the profound depth of Zen, births a potent yet delicate synthesis. While it's paramount to uphold scientific integrity and effective training, there's an equally pressing need to respect and honor the cultural roots of Zen, ensuring its teachings are integrated with sensitivity and reverence.

The narrative of Zen in medicine also illuminates the broader human quest for meaning. Each therapeutic interaction, each medical decision, becomes an avenue for both the patient and healthcare provider to derive deeper meaning, fostering mutual growth and shared enlightenment.

Embracing Zen in this context is not a mere strategy or technique; it's an invitation to a deeper understanding of life, health, and the human spirit. As we venture further into this integration, we don't merely aim for better healthcare outcomes but aspire to elevate the very essence of healthcare itself. Through Zen, we may find the sublime symphony where science, spirit, and humanity converge, creating a holistic paradigm of well-being for the ages.

In the vast realm of medical practice, where science, intuition, and human connection seamlessly intersect, lies a profound approach: the incorporation of Zen principles. "Zen and the Art of Medicine" seeks to delve deep into the heart of how mindfulness, particularly through Zen, can vastly enhance patient care, the well-being of healthcare professionals, and the overall experience of healing.

At the cornerstone of medical care is the doctor-patient relationship. Through cultivating mindfulness, medical practitioners not only elevate the quality of care but also foster a more holistic and empathetic connection with their patients. This enriched perspective aids in the precision of diagnoses and the formulation of effective treatment plans. The intuitive insights drawn from Zen practices open new dimensions, transforming routine medical procedures into profound interactions, filled with compassion and understanding.

Yet, the art of medicine is not just about treating others. Healthcare professionals, often facing the brunt of stress and the overwhelming weight of responsibility, can turn to Zen practices as a sanctuary, reducing burnout and reigniting their passion for healing. Similarly, introducing patients to Zen can revamp rehabilitation programs, making stress management and recovery more holistic. The silent whispers of Zen meditation offer solace, guiding practitioners and patients alike through tumultuous times.

The therapeutic wonders of Zen meditation extend further. From mental domains, where it alleviates the heavy burdens of depression and anxiety and possibly augments cognitive faculties, to physical realms where pain management and immune defense may find a new ally in meditation. Numerous testimonies and emerging research highlight the transformative power of Zen, emphasizing its role in enhancing focus, clarity, and resilience.

Beyond the immediate therapeutic scope, the union of Zen and medicine offers a more preventive and integrative approach to health. Integrating Zen practices daily can be the cornerstone of healthier lifestyles, weaving a protective shield against ailments. This balance of mind and body doesn't just reduce potential health risks but can also diminish the constant reliance on medical interventions. By embracing Zen, individuals can experience a heightened sense of well-being, self-awareness, and harmony. As we delve into the chapters of this book, we will also discover how Zen serves as a harmonious complement to traditional treatments, empowering patients to champion their healing journey alongside their healthcare providers.

As you embark on this enlightening journey through "Zen and the Art of Medicine," prepare to uncover a transformative perspective on healthcare, one that harmoniously blends ancient Zen teachings with modern medical practices. Welcome to a world where medicine is not just a science but an art, refined by the serene principles of Zen and enriched by a deeper understanding of the human experience.

In our ceaseless quest for meaning, we often traverse the vast terrains of human experience. Healthcare, with its intrinsic alignment to the human condition, provides an especially rich tapestry of encounters, emotions, and existential quests. How might Zen, with its timeless wisdom, weave itself into this intricate tapestry, enhancing not just the quality of care, but the very essence of the medical profession?

Within the sanctum of patient-practitioner interactions, there emerges a yearning for genuine connection. When healthcare professionals immerse themselves wholly in the moment, a depth of understanding and heightened discernment unfolds. Such profound presence not only refines diagnostic precision but also rekindles the soulful essence of medicine.

The shadows of burnout and despair, so rampant in healthcare, serve as stark reminders of our existential vacuum. Yet, Zen's teachings shine as a beacon, guiding practitioners away from the abyss of emptiness towards a sanctuary of centeredness. By imbibing this ancient wisdom, both professionals and patients embark on a transformative journey, moving from mere symptom relief to profound spiritual healing.

Zen's meditative practices, though silent and introspective, resonate with profound echoes. For those entrapped in the chains of anxiety or weighed down by depression, Zen offers a lifeline, beckoning mental liberation. Its reverberations touch the physical realm, hinting at alleviated pain and perhaps a fortified immunity. These practices are not mere therapeutic tools; they are gateways to a deeper understanding of our existence.

Wedding Zen's ethereal wisdom with the concrete empiricism of medicine is a delicate dance. It requires rigorous scientific scrutiny, meticulous training, and an unwavering ethical compass. With Zen deeply rooted in the cultural soils of East Asia, its integration demands profound reverence and sensitivity, ensuring that this union respects its origins and avoids the pitfalls of appropriation.

In conclusion, the wedding of Zen and medicine is more than a mere integration; it's an existential exploration. It invites us to see healthcare not just as a means to an end but as a journey filled with meaning, purpose, and profound human connections. Through this lens, we discover that amidst life's challenges and the intricacies of healthcare, there lies an opportunity to heal, discover, and most importantly, to finish.

Moreover, the rejuvenating power of Zen provides a unique sanctuary. Imagine a space where both the healer and the healed find balance and peace. This isn't about eschewing modern medical practices but enriching them. By introducing Zen practices, we not only aid patients but also provide healthcare providers with tools to combat the stresses of their demanding profession.

The therapeutic potential of Zen meditation extends further. Over centuries, this practice has been a beacon of solace and resilience. Now, as we look through the lens of modern healthcare, the implications become even more exciting. There's an emerging awareness of how mental fortitude, cultivated through practices like Zen meditation, can have tangible health benefits.

This journey also nudges us to evaluate the role of Zen in physical well-being. Could ancient Zen techniques offer insights or even solutions to contemporary health challenges? As we explore this, we also venture into the holistic approach Zen brings to preventative healthcare. By emphasizing a harmonious balance between mind and body, Zen might pave the way for reduced dependencies on curative interventions, steering the focus toward prevention.

The integration doesn't stop there. As we anticipate the fusion of Zen principles and modern medicine, the landscape of our healthcare system begins to transform. This is a vision of a system where collaboration, respect, and deep understanding shape patient-provider interactions.

Our journey through the vastness of human experiences uncovers the potent rejuvenation Zen offers. This realm isn't about sidelining modern medical practices; instead, it's about magnifying their essence. Through Zen, we don't only uplift patients but also equip healthcare professionals with resilience against the relentless pressures they face.

The centuries-old practice of Zen meditation stands as a sanctuary of resilience. Gazing through the modern healthcare prism, the potential of mental strength, cultivated through such meditative practices, to yield tangible health dividends becomes clear. This reflection further nudges us to ponder Zen's role in bodily wellness. Could these ancient Zen techniques provide keys to today's health puzzles? Zen's holistic approach, emphasizing mind-body harmony, potentially shifts our gaze from curative actions to preventive measures.

However, this integration isn't just a fusion of two domains; it's a transformation of the entire healthcare vista. It paints a vision of healthcare where deep respect, collaboration, and mutual understanding dictate every patient-provider interaction.

But blending these domains isn't without its intricacies. As we venture down this path, the need for tact, honor, and meticulousness becomes evident. The convergence of Zen and medicine isn't merely the merging of practices but the interlacing of cultures, legacies, and ideologies. Throughout this endeavor, Zen's rich cultural roots must remain in the spotlight, respected and cherished.

To our readers, this narrative intertwines the tranquil essence of Zen with the dynamic terrain of medicine. Whether your interests lie in Zen, healthcare, research, or pure curiosity, there's a wealth of insights waiting. This exploration is tailored to cater to a myriad of readers: from Zen novices seeking foundational insights to healthcare mavens exploring integrative methodologies. We invite every reader to traverse the vast potentials of Zen and medicine, envisioning a future healthcare paradigm rooted in mindfulness and holistic understanding.

As we prepare to delve into the depths of this rich narrative, we aim to facilitate a journey that offers each reader a personalized path through the abundant information housed in this book.

We envision this book serving as a guide, a mentor, and a rich resource, offering a wealth of insights and tools that cater to a diverse array of readers. Join us as we unravel the potential paths one can carve through the extensive tapestry of knowledge, nurturing a deeper understanding and application of Zen in the realm of medicine.

An introduction to the author.

Embarking on a Personal Journey: An Autobiography Deep Rooted in Homeopathic Medicine, astrology and psychology.

Education and Credentials: Building a Foundation at California State Northridge

My educational journey has been significant in shaping my understanding and approach towards holistic health. I earned a master's degree in education with a focus on Psychological Learning at California State Northridge, and have cultivated a rich backdrop that blends the realms of psychology with education, setting a robust foundation for a career deeply intertwined with holistic healing practices.

Decades of Experience: From Patient to Intern to Practitioner

The decades that followed 1980 have seen me evolving through various roles - from being a patient to an intern, and eventually blossoming into a practitioner in the homeopathic field. This period allowed for a rich accumulation of experiences and insights, each role offering a unique perspective and deepening my understanding of homeopathic medicine. Through the autobiography, I share tales from each phase, offering readers a glimpse into the world of homeopathic medicine seen through different lenses.

Through a very thorough and comprehensive self-prescribed regime of homeopathic remedies, I was able to overcome stage four Parkinson's. Stage five is a wheelchair and beyond that is death.

At this point, I have a very thorough and wonderful exercise routine, which consists of yoga, weight training, and swimming. My exercise program extends to seven days a week. I enjoy, listening to music in the morning and dancing in my stocking feet.

An Astrological Perspective: A Published Author in the Field of Astrology with many years of experience in this field.

Adding another layer to my expertise is my venture into the field of astrology. I have authored two books in this field, and bring to the table a depth of understanding that goes beyond the conventional realm of medicine, touching upon the cosmic influences that govern our lives. The autobiography promises an enriching exploration into the intriguing parallels between astrology and homeopathy, offering readers an exhilarating journey across the boundaries of science and the mystical realms of astrological insights.

A Voice in the Digital Age: Sharing Wisdom Through Social Media

In recent years, my endeavor to share knowledge and insights took a digital turn as I began to leverage various social media platforms. Through numerous articles focused on holistic medicine, psychology, and homeopathic practices, I have engaged with a global audience, fostering a space of learning and discourse. This autobiography encapsulates the wisdom distilled from these articles, offering readers a consolidated space to engage with a rich tapestry of insights garnered over years of exploration and practice.

As we stand at the threshold of this autobiographical narrative, I extend a warm invitation to readers to join me on this introspective journey that promises not just a recounting of personal experiences but a deep dive into the holistic world of homeopathic medicine and astrology.

It is a narrative that goes beyond a mere autobiography, bringing forth a rich blend of professional insights, educational pursuits, and a profound understanding of the cosmic and psychological dimensions that govern the realm of holistic health. Join me as I unfold a journey spanning over four decades, sharing the richness and depth of experiences that have shaped my understanding and practice in the fields of homeopathic medicine and astrology.

Setting the Stage for a Profound Journey Through Zen and Medicine

As we approach the conclusion of this introductory segment, it is pertinent to underscore the rich tapestry of knowledge and insights that await you in the forthcoming chapters of this seminal book on Zen and medicine. The journey we are about to undertake is both deep and extensive, rooted in a profound understanding of Zen principles and their intricate relationships with various facets of medicine.

As we begin this exploration, let's appreciate the vast ocean of knowledge awaiting us in this unique intersection of Zen and medicine. We're about to dive deep, exploring the profound essence of Zen and its intricate relationship with medicine's multifaceted world.

Chapter 1: The Convergence of Zen and Medicine

The Philosophical Foundations of Zen

Core beliefs of Zen Buddhism

Zen Buddhism is deeply entrenched in the doctrines established by the Mahayana school of Buddhism, placing a heavy emphasis on meditation and the personal pursuit of enlightenment. While other forms of Buddhism often focus on the study of scriptures and the following of specific rites and rituals, Zen Buddhism argues that these are secondary, encouraging its practitioners to engage in meditation (Zazen) and to perceive the natural world directly. This concept is rooted in the inherent Buddha nature of all beings and the belief that enlightenment can be achieved by anyone.

One of the central beliefs in Zen is the concept of "Kensho" which refers to the direct perception or insight into one's true nature. Additionally, the school of Zen is known for its non-reliance on written scriptures, preferring transmission through direct communication and teachings from master to student, fostering a personal and direct approach to spirituality.

Understanding the Four Noble Truths

The Four Noble Truths are essentially the cornerstone of Buddhism, acting as the foundation upon which all teachings and practices are built.

Suffering (Dukkha): Suffering is a part of human life, and it arises from various sources including physical pain, separation from loved ones, and not getting what one desires. Suffering is inherent to life's impermanence, where even joyful moments are tinged with the knowledge that they will end.

Origin of Suffering (Samudaya): This Noble Truth looks at the cause of suffering, largely rooted in desire and ignorance. The teachings encourage individuals to understand the roots of their desires and the resulting suffering to be able to alleviate them.

Cessation of Suffering (Nirodha): Here, it's taught that it is possible to end suffering by relinquishing attachment and desire. This cessation is referred to as "Nirvana", a state of liberation and freedom from suffering.

Path to the Cessation of Suffering (Magga): This truth outlines the path that leads to the end of suffering, known as the Noble Eightfold Path. It comprises moral principles and practices that guide individuals to live a life of moderation and ethical conduct, fostering wisdom and meditation practices.

The Noble Eightfold Path: Guiding Principles to End Suffering

Right Understanding (Sammā-diṭṭhi): This pertains to the understanding of things as they truly are. It means grasping the Four Noble Truths and understanding the nature of the self and the world.

Right Intention (Sammā-saṅkappa): This involves the cultivation of compassion and loving-kindness, as well as the absence of cruelty, ill-will, and desire. It means deciding to act and think without harming oneself or others.

Right Speech (Sammā-vācā): Abstaining from lying, divisive speech, harsh words, and idle chatter. Instead, one should speak the truth, and be harmonious, gentle, and meaningful.

Right Action (Sammā-kammanta): Refraining from harmful behaviors, such as taking life, stealing, and engaging in sexual misconduct. This path element encourages moral and honorable actions.

Right Livelihood (Sammā-ājīva): Ensuring one's profession doesn't harm oneself or others. Examples of jobs to avoid include those that involve killing (like weapon selling) or that exploit others.

Right Effort (Sammā-vāyāma): Cultivating and maintaining wholesome qualities while avoiding and getting rid of unwholesome ones. It means to generate enthusiasm, desire, effort, diligence, and perseverance in maintaining beneficial states of mind.

Right Mindfulness (Sammā-sati): This is the continuous and clear awareness of one's body actions, feelings, sensations, and mind states. It involves being fully present and attentive to experiences, without being reactive or distracted.

Right Concentration (Sammā-samādhi): Developing the mental focus necessary for deep meditation. This can lead to the jhanas, which are advanced states of concentration. Right concentration is about cultivating a unified, focused mind.

In Zen Buddhism, the concept of non-self, or "anatta", dictates that the perception of one's self is not rooted in a permanent, unchanging entity, but is a construct formed through a complex interplay of elements that are continuously changing. This philosophical approach challenges the inherent belief systems about personal identity, urging individuals to explore the transient nature of existence.

In Zen practice, understanding the self goes beyond superficial layers of identity, delving deep into one's mind and consciousness through meditation and mindfulness. The approach seeks to strip away ego and superficial perceptions to arrive at a state of pure awareness, a realization of the interconnectedness of all things and the transient nature of all phenomena.

Zen promotes the notion of holistic health, advocating for a deep interconnectedness between the mind and the body. By nurturing a deep understanding of the self through practices like meditation and heightened awareness, practitioners can promote mental clarity, reduce stress, and foster a sense of well-being. It also encourages practitioners to cultivate a healthy lifestyle through balanced nutrition, physical activity, and harmonious living with nature and others. This mind-body integration in medicine also is reflected in the practice of homeopathic medicine.

The historical origins and developments of Buddhism expanded

Zen Buddhism initially developed as a school of Mahayana Buddhism in China during the 6th century CE. The initial development period saw the integration of several Chinese philosophies, including Taoism and Confucianism, which profoundly influenced its character, making it a unique school of thought focusing on the individual's direct experience and personal enlightenment.

Zen Buddhism can trace its philosophical roots back to the Indian subcontinent, originating from the teachings of Siddhartha Gautama, who later became known as Buddha. Over time, these teachings were carried over into China, melding with the local philosophies and cultural nuances to birth Chan Buddhism, a precursor to Zen.

While Zen Buddhism entered Japan around the 7th century, it wasn't until the 12th century that it started flourishing. Over time, distinct schools within Zen Buddhism emerged, including the Rinzai and Soto schools, each having its emphasis — the Rinzai on Koan study and the Soto on seated meditation or "Zazen."

Throughout its history, several figures have stood out in the Zen tradition. Bodhidharma, credited with being the founder of Zen Buddhism in China, emphasized meditation and direct experience over theoretical knowledge. Dogen, a prominent Japanese Zen master, founded the Soto school, emphasizing "shikantaza," or "just sitting." Meanwhile, Eisai, another critical figure, introduced the Rinzai school to Japan, a school that makes significant use of "Koans," paradoxical anecdotes or riddles, as a meditation discipline to provoke doubt and test one's progress.

Zen masters

Bodhidharma: This semi-legendary figure is considered the first patriarch of Zen, emphasizing a meditation-based practice termed "wall-gazing." His focus was to bring people back to a meditation-based practice and personal enlightenment.

Dogen: Dogen is credited with bringing Soto Zen from China to Japan, fostering the "Shikantaza" or "just sitting" meditation technique. His teachings have been compiled in extensive written works, including the Shōbōgenzō, a collection of 95 essays on Buddhist practice and teachings.

Hakuin Ekaku: A pivotal figure in the Rinzai school of Zen, Hakuin revitalized the tradition, focusing extensively on Koan practice. He is known for his calligraphic artworks and paintings, which were also a part of his teaching method, using them as visual expressions of Zen concepts.

Understanding the deep roots and vast spectrum of philosophies within Zen Buddhism offers a profound and rich perspective on its practices and the underpinning philosophies guiding its teachings. It is a pathway that encourages self-discovery, deep awareness, and a harmonious existence with all of existence, advocating a practice that goes beyond mere intellectual understanding to a deeper, experiential comprehension of the self and the universe.

What follows is a Journey into the Understanding, of holistic, medicine, its principles, and practices.

Holistic medicine revolves around a healing approach that considers the whole person—body, mind, spirit, and emotions—in the quest for optimal health and wellness. The core belief is that, for optimal health to be achieved, one must gain proper balance in life. Practitioners of holistic medicine employ various forms of healthcare practices, including conventional medication and alternative therapies, to prevent and treat diseases, and more importantly, to promote optimal health. It operates on the premise that the body can heal itself if given the right support.

Central to holistic medicine is the approach of treating the individual in their entirety rather than just focusing on the disease. This involves understanding and addressing the underlying causes of the disease, not just alleviating symptoms. It encompasses a deeper understanding of a patient's history, emotional well-being, lifestyle, and other elements to formulate a treatment plan that is specially tailored to the individual, thereby fostering more effective healing and wellness.

Integrative medicine represents a harmonization of Western and Eastern approaches to medicine, bringing together the best of both worlds for a more comprehensive approach to health care. In this approach, innovative medical techniques are combined with traditional practices, such as acupuncture, yoga, herbal medicine, and homeopathic medicine, to create a healthcare plan that works holistically. The aim is to treat not just the body, but also the mind and spirit, to foster overall well-being.

A holistic approach to medicine has a wide range of benefits, including, a greater focus on prevention and lifestyle improvements, and the potential to discover and treat the root cause of an illness rather than just managing symptoms. Furthermore, it promotes the idea of self-care, empowering individuals to take charge of their health.

By focusing on the individual as a whole, a holistic approach often leads to better patient outcomes. It encourages lifestyle changes that are more sustainable in the long run, helping patients manage their health conditions more effectively and potentially reducing the need for medical interventions. Moreover, encouraging a stronger patient-practitioner relationship fosters a more collaborative and empowering healthcare experience.

Historically, Zen Buddhism and its principles have been integrated into medical practices. Early on, Zen monks were known to be healers, utilizing various herbs and acupuncture in treatments. They integrated a holistic approach to healing, which considered the well-being of the mind and the body interconnected.

Modern-day scenario

In contemporary medicine, there is a resurgence of Zen principles, with many practitioners recognizing the benefits of a more holistic approach to health and well-being. This approach advocates for preventative measures such as meditation and yoga to maintain a healthy balance between mind and body, offering a more rounded approach to health care that recognizes the interconnectedness of all aspects of an individual's health. This resurgence reflects a growing understanding of the deep interconnection between mind and body, and the importance of maintaining a harmonious balance for overall health and well-being. It brings back the focus on personal enlightenment and inner peace as central components in achieving overall health.

Holistic medicine including some contemporary approaches, Chinese, East Indian, and homeopathic medicine operates with a patient-centered philosophy, positing that individuals are not merely a sum of their parts or defined by the diseases or conditions they have. This approach encourages healthcare providers to engage deeply with patients, understanding their personal histories, environments, and lifestyles to tailor a treatment strategy that addresses the root causes of their ailments, rather than just the symptoms.

Considering factors such as a person's mental health, social factors, and physical conditions, the holistic approach seeks to restore balance and health in the most natural way possible. It may involve incorporating psychological therapy to address mental health concerns or prescribing dietary changes to foster physical health. The strategy might also recognize and attempt to mitigate environmental factors contributing to the individual's health condition. By embracing this philosophy, practitioners foster a nurturing and trusting relationship with their patients, which in turn can create a supportive atmosphere that is conducive to healing and well-being.

Through this kind of individual-centered approach, patients are often endowed with a greater understanding and awareness of their bodies and health conditions, fostering autonomy and encouraging proactive engagement with their health.

Integrative medicine stands as a testament to the harmonious blending of Eastern and Western medicinal approaches, creating a more rounded and comprehensive healthcare paradigm that seeks to promote optimal health by considering the individual as a whole—encompassing mind, body, and spirit. This method is increasingly gaining traction in the contemporary healthcare landscape, as it brings a multidimensional approach to treatment that caters to all facets of an individual's well-being.

One of the remarkable aspects of integrative medicine is its flexibility and adaptability, allowing for a broad spectrum of therapies to be utilized. For instance, a patient undergoing treatment for chronic pain might be offered a combination of pharmaceutical treatments, acupuncture, physical therapy, and mindfulness meditation as part of their treatment plan. They may also be introduced to the benefits of homeopathic prescribing. Acupuncture and meditation, drawing from Eastern traditions, could offer complementary benefits to Western medical treatments, fostering a holistic healing environment that addresses both the physical symptoms and the psychological or spiritual dimensions of the pain.

By incorporating treatments like yoga and herbal and homeopathic medicine, it seeks to foster well-being not just through alleviating physical symptoms, but also by promoting mental peace and spiritual harmony. These forms of medicine recognize the interconnectedness of different aspects of individual health and operate on the understanding that addressing one facet in isolation might not yield the desired results.

In essence, the cultural integration of Western and Eastern, processing medicine, brings together the scientific advancements and the technological prowess of the Western paradigm with the time-honored, holistic approaches of Eastern medicine, to work toward a common goal of achieving optimal health and wellness. It's a harmonious amalgamation of philosophies that leverages the strengths and addresses the limitations of both systems to create a more effective healthcare strategy.

One of the core principles of integrative medicine is its emphasis on the doctor-patient relationship. It fosters a collaborative environment where the patient is actively involved in their healthcare decisions, working hand in hand with the practitioner. This involves an open dialogue where both parties communicate freely and openly, fostering trust and understanding.

As previously outlined, homeopathic prescribing can be a very helpful adjunct to conventional medications and treatments

Nutritional therapy is another crucial aspect, drawing from the Eastern focus on diet as a fundamental element of health. The die factor was also echoed in the teachings of Hippocrates. Integrative practitioners may work closely with individuals to develop nutrition plans that support health and prevent disease, recognizing the significant role that diet plays in overall wellness

.

Nutritional therapy is a therapeutic approach that utilizes the science of nutrition and dietary choices to promote health, manage health conditions, and support overall well-being. It is often guided by trained nutritional therapists or registered dietitians who work with individuals to develop personalized dietary plans.

Core Principles of Nutritional Therapy:

Diet-Health Connection: It recognizes the profound impact of diet on physical and mental health, with an emphasis on the importance of a balanced diet.

Individualized Approach: Nutritional therapists assess each client's unique needs, considering factors such as age, lifestyle, medical history, and dietary preferences.

Evidence-Based Practice: Recommendations are based on scientific research and nutritional guidelines.

The Role of the Nutritional Therapist:

Trained nutritional therapists assess clients' nutritional status and health goals.

They develop personalized dietary plans, guiding food choices, portion control, and meal timing.

Dietary Components:

Nutritional therapy encompasses various dietary components, including macronutrients (carbohydrates, proteins, and fats), micronutrients (vitamins and minerals), and dietary fiber.

Specialized diets, such as gluten-free or ketogenic diets, may be recommended based on individual needs.

Vitamins and Minerals:

Vitamin A: Supports healthy vision, immune function, and skin health. Found in sweet potatoes, carrots, and leafy greens.

Vitamin C: Boosts the immune system, aids in collagen production, and acts as a powerful antioxidant. Found in citrus fruits, strawberries, and bell peppers.

Vitamin D: Essential for bone health and immune function. Natural sources include sunlight, and it can also be found in fatty fish like salmon and fortified dairy products.

Vitamin E: An antioxidant that protects cells from damage. Found in nuts, seeds, and vegetable oils.

Vitamin K: Important for blood clotting and bone health. Present in leafy greens like kale and spinach.

Calcium: Crucial for bone health and muscle function. Dairy products, leafy greens, and fortified foods are good sources.

Iron: Essential for oxygen transport in the blood. Found in red meat, beans, and fortified cereals.

Magnesium: Supports muscle and nerve function, bone health, and energy production. Available in nuts, whole grains, and leafy greens.

Zinc: Important for immune function and wound healing. Found in meat, seafood, and legumes.

Nutrient-Dense Foods:

Berries: Rich in antioxidants, fiber, and vitamins. Blueberries, strawberries, and raspberries are great choices.

Leafy Greens: Packed with vitamins, minerals, and fiber. Spinach, kale, and Swiss chard are excellent options.

Fatty Fish: High in omega-3 fatty acids, which support heart and brain health. Include salmon, mackerel, and sardines in your diet.

Nuts and Seeds: Provide healthy fats, protein, and various vitamins and minerals. Almonds, walnuts, and flaxseeds are nutritious choices.

Whole Grains: Rich in fiber and essential nutrients. Opt for whole wheat, oats, quinoa, and brown rice.

Legumes: A great source of plant-based protein, fiber, and various vitamins and minerals. Include beans, lentils, and chickpeas in your meals.

Yogurt: Contains probiotics for gut health and is a good source of calcium and protein. Choose plain, unsweetened yogurt.

Colorful Vegetables: A variety of vegetables, such as carrots, bell peppers, and sweet potatoes, provide an array of vitamins and antioxidants.

Lean Proteins: Chicken, turkey, lean cuts of beef, and tofu offer protein with minimal saturated fat.

Herbs and Spices: Add flavor and health benefits. Turmeric, garlic, and cinnamon have anti-inflammatory properties.

In the realm of wellness centers, nutritional therapy is an essential component of promoting well-being. It's a personalized and science-backed approach to enhance overall health and vitality, utilizing a wide array of nutrient-rich foods and essential vitamins and minerals. Nutritional therapists tailor recommendations based on individual needs and health objectives, aiming to support wellness and long-term health.

Populations and Settings:

Nutritional therapy can benefit individuals of all ages, from children to seniors, and is relevant in various settings, including clinical, community, and sports nutrition.

In a clinical setting, it may be used to manage chronic diseases like diabetes or support weight management.

Goals of Nutritional Therapy:

Nutritional therapy aims to achieve various health-related goals, such as weight management, blood sugar control, improved digestion, and enhanced energy levels.

In an athletic context, it can optimize performance and recovery through appropriate nutrition.

Assessment and Evaluation:

Nutritional therapists assess clients' dietary habits, conduct nutritional analyses, and monitor progress.

Regular check-ins and adjustments to the dietary plan are common to track improvements or address challenges.

Ethical Considerations:

Nutritional therapists adhere to ethical standards, ensuring client confidentiality, cultural sensitivity, and responsible dietary advice.

In the context of nutritional therapy, clients receive personalized guidance on making dietary choices that align with their health goals. This approach can help individuals achieve better health, manage chronic conditions, and enjoy a higher quality of life through evidence-based nutritional recommendations tailored to their unique needs.

In conclusion, integrative medicine stands as a beacon of balanced healthcare, harmonizing the technological advancements of Western medicine with the holistic, person-centered philosophies of Eastern healthcare traditions. It's an approach that doesn't just aim to treat diseases but to promote overall well-being, recognizing the interdependent relationship between mind, body, and spirit and fostering health through a multidimensional, collaborative, and deeply personal approach to healthcare. It is a domain continuously evolving, adapting to discoveries and knowledge while retaining the age-old wisdom from diverse medical traditions, to cater to the unique needs of every individual and ensure a state of complete physical, mental, and social well-being.

A deeper exploration into the Early incorporations of Zen in medicine and the role that early Zen monks and monasteries played in the proliferation of his approach to medicine

In the early stages of its incorporation into medicine, Zen Buddhism played a vital role in influencing the healthcare approaches during those periods. This was deeply rooted in its philosophies concerning the interconnectedness of mind and body and the focus on holistic well-being rather than just the treatment of diseases. The Zen approach to health often involved a holistic assessment of the individual, encompassing physical, mental, and even spiritual aspects.

In the United States, for instance, the integration of meditation has seen a steady increase. It is being employed in various clinical settings to aid in stress reduction, improve mental health, and enhance overall well-being. Initiatives like the Mindfulness-Based Stress Reduction (MBSR) program have gained prominence, offering structured training in mindfulness meditation to help individuals manage chronic pain, anxiety, depression, and other health issues.

Meanwhile, in Japan, a country with a rich Zen Buddhist history, we observe the practice of "Shinrin-yoku" or forest bathing, a concept deeply aligned with Zen principles of harmonizing oneself with nature, which has been recognized for its therapeutic potential. This practice encourages individuals to immerse themselves in forest environments to foster mental tranquility and enhance well-being, drawing upon the Zen idea of being one with nature to facilitate healing.

It promotes mindfully connecting with nature to experience its calming and healing benefits. This practice isn't about physical bathing but centers on mental and emotional rejuvenation from spending time in a forest.

Examples of places worldwide utilizing forest bathing include Japan, which is recognized as the birthplace of Shinrin-yoku and has meticulously crafted forest therapy trails. The ethereal beauty of Yakushima Island, with its moss-covered ancient trees, and the majestic landscapes of the Japanese Alps, make them top destinations for immersive forest experiences.

In South Korea, Jeju Island is renowned not just for its stunning beaches but also for its Healing Forest Center, a testament to the country's dedication to forest therapy.

Both the colossal redwoods of Muir Woods National Monument in California and the sprawling landscapes of the Great Smoky Mountains in Tennessee are iconic American sites for forest bathing.

The Ancient Forest Alliance in British Columbia, Canada, is a testament to the country's commitment to connecting humans with age-old trees.

The rugged beauty of the Scottish Highlands offers an authentic and tranquil forest therapy experience.

Community Healing Circles are therapeutic gatherings where people come together in a supportive setting. Here, they share experiences, emotions, and stories. The circles prioritize active listening, empathy, and collective support. They aim to encourage healing, resilience, and community bonding.

In the United States, New York City's Center for Court Innovation pioneers in merging traditional legal procedures with restorative justice practices.

Canada's Indigenous communities historically use healing circles as an ancestral tradition.

Post-apartheid South Africa saw the Truth and Reconciliation Commission hearings serve as a balm, incorporating elements of healing circles.

Australia's Aboriginal and Torres Strait Islander communities use "yarning circles" for sharing stories and healing.

In Northern Ireland, healing circles have become integral to peace and reconciliation efforts.

Set amidst the verdant landscapes of Neyyar Dam, Kerala, Sivananda Ashram doesn't just offer yoga and meditation retreats; it provides a holistic journey.

Osho International Meditation Resort in Pune stands apart for its modern approach to meditation, blending spirituality and luxury.

The spiritual city of Rishikesh houses the Parmarth Niketan Ashram, offering transformative experiences on the banks of the Ganges River.

Vipassana Meditation Retreats, scattered across India, are renowned for their rigorous approach, emphasizing deep introspection.

In the pristine landscapes of Coimbatore lies the Isha Yoga Center, offering unique meditation forms amidst breathtaking natural beauty.

Nestled in the serene McLeod Ganj region of Dharamshala, the Tushita Meditation Center stands as a spiritual sanctuary.

Amidst the cultural richness of Chiang Mai, Wat Rampoeng stands as a beacon for those seeking inner peace, guiding practitioners in mindfulness and Vipassana meditation.

Wat Umong in Chiang Mai is famed for its ancient tunnels and forested surroundings, offering a unique meditation experience.

Right in the heart of Bangkok, Suanthip serves as a sanctuary from the urban hustle, offering an oasis of calm for Vipassana practitioners.

Not far from Bangkok, the Wat Phra Dhammakaya complex stands as a symbol of modern Buddhism, emphasizing the Dhammakaya meditation technique.

Located in Southern Thailand, Wat Suan Mokkh offers intensive 10-day silent meditation retreats, fostering deeper understanding and self-awareness.

Each of these practices and retreats, while rooted in unique traditions and methods, share a common goal: guiding individuals toward inner peace, self-realization, and a deeper connection with the surrounding world. They serve as sanctuaries for the soul, providing paths to holistic well-being and enlightenment.

In the context of Europe, countries like the UK and Germany have been exploring and accepting meditation techniques as complementary practices in healthcare settings. These practices, rooted in Zen principles, are used as supportive therapies in mental health treatments, helping individuals cope with stress, anxiety, and depressive symptoms, demonstrating the universal applicability and benefit of these Zen-inspired practices.

Beyond clinical settings, there has been a rise in the acceptance and practice of yoga and meditation in daily lives, across cultures and countries, embracing the Zen philosophy of nurturing the mind-body connection to foster health and well-being.

Moreover, there has been a renewed interest in herbal and homeopathic medicine, practices that find resonance with the Zen approach to healing through nature, where countries like China and India are witnessing a revival of traditional herbal and homeopathic medicine practices, with individuals increasingly seeking natural remedies for common ailments. This is especially true in India, which has a vast amount of homeopathic practitioners and clinics available to everyone.

Furthermore, modern healthcare has also seen a trend where more people are inclined towards individualized treatment plans, a concept echoing the Zen principle of seeing and treating the individual as a whole. This not only facilitates a more personalized approach to healthcare but also fosters a nurturing and understanding healthcare environment that promotes collaborative decision-making and encourages individuals to play an active role in their healing journey.

As we delve deeper into the 21st century, the resurgence of Zen principles in modern medicine continues to shape healthcare philosophies and practices globally. It is a reflection of a growing understanding and recognition of the interconnectedness of the mind, body, and spirit, and a testimony to the timeless relevance and universal applicability of Zen philosophies in promoting holistic health and well-being. This resurgence is not just a return to ancient wisdom but a progressive stride towards a more comprehensive, inclusive, and humane approach to healthcare, one that recognizes the individual as a complex interplay of various dimensions working in harmony, necessitating a holistic approach to health and healing. It showcases the evolving landscape of modern healthcare, a fusion of scientific advancements and age-old wisdom, walking hand in hand to create a healthcare future that is holistic, inclusive, and nurturing.

Case Studies: Zen Principles in Healing Practices

As we have witnessed previously, In recent years, the healthcare sector has been encouraging the trend where Zen principles are being adopted to foster more holistic healing experiences. These principles, deeply rooted in mindfulness and interconnectedness of the mind and body, have found expression in various therapeutic practices globally. Through an extensive exploration of case studies, we uncover the profound impact of Zen-inspired healing in real-world scenarios.

Across different continents, there has been a notable increase in the incorporation of Zen principles in therapeutic practices.

United States: Various healthcare centers have initiated programs such as Zen art therapy where patients are encouraged to immerse themselves in artistic endeavors, finding a calm and focused state of mind, which is integral in recovery paths, especially for individuals dealing with trauma or mental health issues.

Art therapy is more than just creating art; it's a bridge between emotional challenges and their expression. Rooted in the idea that creative expression can unlock emotional hurdles, art therapy aids individuals in exploring feelings that may not easily be verbalized. From the depths of traumatic experiences to the heights of personal successes, art provides a canvas for the soul's narratives.

While the therapeutic process is deeply personal, trained art therapists play an essential role. They're not just observers; they're guides, navigating the therapeutic journey alongside their clients. Their training, which melds therapeutic practice with artistic understanding, enables them to suggest techniques and mediums that best suit an individual's therapeutic needs. For instance, while some might find solace in the brush strokes of painting, others might resonate more with molding clay or crafting a collage.

Art therapy's applications are vast. Beyond individual therapy, it has shown promise in group settings, promoting community bonding and collective healing. Schools, rehabilitation centers, and even prisons have employed art therapy to address issues like anxiety, interpersonal challenges, and self-esteem.

Art therapy is a therapeutic approach that uses the creation and exploration of visual art forms as a means of self-expression, communication, and healing. It is often facilitated by trained art therapists who help individuals, groups, or communities engage in the artistic process to address emotional, psychological, or physical challenges.

What also can be of great benefit, is Music therapy, similarly, which has a profound impact on the human psyche. It isn't merely about listening to or playing music. It's about harnessing the universal language of melodies, rhythms, and harmonies to heal. Music can transport us—to memories long forgotten or to feelings left unexplored.

Music therapists, equipped with knowledge in both therapeutic and musical domains, curate personalized experiences for their clients. For a child with autism, rhythmic drumming might foster social connection. For a stroke survivor, singing might aid speech recovery. Even in neonatal units, lullabies have been used to soothe premature infants, promoting essential weight gain and growth.

Music Therapy: An Overview

Definition: Music therapy is the use of musical interventions to accomplish individualized goals within a therapeutic relationship by a credentialed professional. This therapeutic form has ancient roots, but its modern practice began in the 20th century, particularly after World Wars I and II, when musicians played for war veterans suffering from physical and emotional trauma.

Global Organizations Promoting Music Therapy:

One notable organization is the American Music Therapy Association (AMTA). Founded in 1998, AMTA promotes the advancement of music therapy practice, research, and education. Similarly, other countries have their respective organizations, such as the British Association for Music Therapy in the UK and the Australian Music Therapy Association in Australia.

Applications in Pain Management:

Distraction: Engaging in music can divert the patient's attention from pain. Music serves as an external stimulus, shifting the focus from internal discomfort to the external auditory experience.

Relaxation: Slow-tempo and rhythmic music can promote relaxation, reducing muscle tension and pain. The predictability of certain rhythms and melodies can help individuals synchronize their breathing and heart rate, leading to a deeper state of calm.

Endorphin release: Music can stimulate the release of endorphins, the body's natural painkillers. The emotional connection to certain songs or melodies can trigger a sense of euphoria, thus helping in pain reduction.

Applications in Spectrum Disorder (e.g., Autism):

Improving Communication: Music therapy can help improve non-verbal and verbal communication skills. Melodic intonation therapy, for instance, utilizes musical elements to improve speech capabilities, especially in those who have lost their ability to speak following brain injuries or conditions like stroke.

Emotional Expression: Music provides a non-threatening medium for individuals to express their feelings. For those with difficulties in traditional communication, musical instruments can serve as an alternative voice, allowing for a full range of emotional expression.

Social Interaction: Group music therapy sessions can enhance social interaction skills. By playing instruments together or engaging in group singing, individuals can connect, practicing essential social cues and building relationships.

Successes in Music Therapy:

In general, music therapy has shown remarkable success in improving the quality of life, reducing symptoms of anxiety and depression, and enhancing cognitive and motor skills among diverse populations.

Dementia Care: Music therapy has been particularly effective for individuals with dementia. It can evoke memories, reduce agitation, improve mood, zend enhance cognitive function. Personalized music playlists, for example, have been shown to reignite memories and bring moments of clarity to dementia patients.

Stroke Rehabilitation: For stroke survivors, music therapy can aid in motor rehabilitation, improving gait and arm strength. Additionally, it can enhance speech and language skills for those with aphasia, a common post-stroke condition.

Alpha and Beta Brainwave Frequencies:

Alpha Waves (8-14 Hz):

Associated with relaxed alertness and calmness, these waves are often dominant when the mind is free from stress and is in a meditative state. They play a crucial role in mental coordination, calmness, alertness, and learning.

Facilitates stress reduction, meditation, and creativity. When alpha waves dominate, it becomes easier for individuals to delve into creative tasks, as they can tap into a more intuitive state of mind.

Applications:

Breathing and Heart Rate Regulation: Inducing alpha wave states can promote a relaxed rhythm in breathing and heart rate, beneficial for stress relief and meditative practices.

Motor Rehabilitation: The relaxation properties of alpha waves can aid in the relaxation of muscles, making it easier to retrain motor functions, especially after an injury.

Speech and Communication: Enhancing alpha states can improve focus and attention, aiding in communication therapies, especially for those with attention-related disorders.

Beta Waves (14-30 Hz):

Associated with active, analytical thought and problem-solving, beta waves dominate our normal waking state when we are attentive and engaged in mental activities.

Applications:

Cognitive Tasks: Enhancing beta wave states can improve performance in tasks that require active thinking, such as problem-solving or decision-making.

Stimulation: Beta waves can be useful in situations where alertness and attention are needed, such as during examinations or critical thinking exercises.

Integration of Brainwave Frequencies in Music Therapy:

Targeted Music Selection: Therapists can select music with rhythms and tempos that align with desired brainwave states, customizing therapeutic interventions for individual needs.

Binaural Beats: This involves playing two slightly different frequencies in each ear. The brain perceives a third tone that's the mathematical difference between the two. It's believed that binaural beats can enhance the production of the desired brainwave states, aiding in relaxation or focus, depending on the frequency difference.

Feedback Mechanisms: Some therapies involve real-time monitoring of brainwaves, and adjusting musical inputs to achieve the desired state. This technique can be especially beneficial for those with disorders affecting brainwave patterns, offering a tailored therapeutic experience.

Remember, while music therapy has demonstrated benefits in various areas, it's essential to consult with professionals to determine its appropriateness and specific applications for each individual. This ensures that the interventions align with the unique needs and conditions of the individual, optimizing therapeutic outcomes.

Music Therapy: Further Insights

The brain processes music in a complex, multifaceted manner, engaging regions responsible for auditory processing, emotion, memory, and more. This wide engagement of brain areas explains why music can have profound effects on our cognition, emotion, and even physical functions.

Neuroplasticity and Music: One of the brain's incredible properties is its ability to change and adapt. This phenomenon, known as neuroplasticity, is at the forefront of why music therapy can be so impactful. By consistently engaging the brain with music, it's possible to strengthen neural connections and even form new ones, potentially aiding recovery after a brain injury or in conditions like dementia.

Applications in Pediatric Care:

Developmental Support: For children with developmental delays or disabilities, music therapy offers an avenue to improve motor skills, cognitive function, and emotional development. Instruments, for example, can be used to improve fine motor skills, while group music sessions can enhance social interaction.

Emotional Well-being: Children, especially those in hospital settings or with chronic conditions, can benefit emotionally from music therapy. It can serve as an emotional outlet, a source of comfort, and a means to express feelings they might not otherwise articulate.

Applications in Mental Health:

Depression and Anxiety: Engaging in music therapy sessions has shown promise in reducing symptoms of depression and anxiety. Creating, listening to, or moving to music can serve as a distraction from negative thoughts, evoke positive emotions, and provide a sense of accomplishment.

Post-traumatic Stress Disorder (PTSD): Music therapy can offer a safe space for trauma survivors to explore and express their emotions, aiding in processing traumatic events and alleviating associated symptoms.

Future Directions and Challenges:

While the benefits of music therapy are becoming increasingly recognized, there are challenges to its widespread adoption. One such challenge is the need for more comprehensive, large-scale studies to solidify its efficacy across various conditions. Furthermore, access to trained music therapists is limited in many areas, making it essential to expand educational and training programs in this field.

In the future, with the integration of technology, we might see innovative approaches like virtual reality-based music therapy or

AI-driven personalized music interventions, which can tailor the therapeutic experience to each individual's needs.

Conclusively, music therapy's interdisciplinary nature, encompassing aspects of neuroscience, psychology, and the arts, gives it a unique position in the therapeutic landscape. As research continues and awareness grows, it holds the promise of unlocking further healing potential for myriad conditions and individuals.

The potential therapeutic applications are as diverse as the music genres themselves. Guided imagery and music (GIM), for instance, involves listening to specific music pieces to evoke imagery and emotions, facilitating introspection and understanding. Neurologic music therapy, on the other hand, harnesses musical elements to address specific cognitive, sensory, and motor dysfunctions.

Furthermore, the positive effects of music therapy are increasingly being validated through scientific research. Brain imaging studies, for instance, have shown that music can activate regions in the brain associated with memory, emotion, and even motor function. This has led to its integration into rehabilitative care, especially for individuals recovering from traumatic brain injuries or strokes.

In conclusion, both art and music therapy stand as testaments to the power of creative expression. They remind us that healing isn't just a clinical process—it can be an artistic journey. By delving into these therapeutic avenues, we unlock doors to self-understanding, resilience, and holistic well-being. Whether through the colors of a canvas or the notes of a melody, art and music therapy offer transformative experiences, blending creativity with healing in symphonies of self-discovery.

South Korea: Zen principles have been integrated into rehabilitation programs for individuals recovering from surgeries, leveraging meditation techniques to foster faster and more holistic recovery.

As we delve deeper into experiences emanating from Zen-inspired healing, we find a rich canvas of therapies including, but not limited to:

Meditation Retreats: Places like Thailand and India have seen a surge in meditation retreats, which offer a sanctuary for individuals to immerse themselves in deep healing through meditation and other Zen practices.

Forest Therapy: This form of therapy, notably practiced in Japan, offers individuals a tranquil space to reconnect with nature and themselves, fostering a nurturing environment for healing.

Introduction to Forest Bathing:

Forest bathing, known as "Shinrin-yoku" in Japanese, is a therapeutic practice rooted in the profound connection between humans and nature. It is a simple yet powerful way to immerse oneself in the natural world, allowing for physical, mental, and emotional rejuvenation through mindful engagement with forests and woodlands. While it does not involve physical bathing, it offers a refreshing "bath" of the senses, where one absorbs the sights, sounds, and scents of the forest environment.

The Concept and Origins:

The concept of forest bathing was developed in Japan in the 1980s as a response to the stress and disconnection from nature often associated with modern urban living. It draws inspiration from ancient Shinto and Buddhist practices that emphasized the healing properties of nature and the importance of harmony between humans and the environment. Today, it has evolved into a recognized form of nature therapy with proven health benefits.

Benefits of Forest Bathing:

Forest bathing offers a multitude of physical, mental, and emotional benefits, making it a valuable practice for overall well-being:

• Stress Reduction: Spending time in nature, particularly forests, has been shown to reduce stress hormone levels, lower blood pressure, and induce a state of relaxation. The calming atmosphere of the forest aids in stress relief.

• Enhanced Mood: Forest bathing is known to improve mood and emotional well-being. The natural environment stimulates the release of endorphins, the brain's "feel-good" chemicals, leading to a sense of happiness and contentment.

• Improved Immune Function: Phytoncides, natural compounds released by trees and plants, have been linked to enhanced immune system activity. Breathing in these substances during forest bathing may boost immune function.

• Increased Focus and Creativity: Time in nature has been associated with improved attention spans, creativity, and problem-solving abilities. It provides a mental break from the demands of modern life.

• Better Sleep: Regular forest bathing can contribute to better sleep quality. Exposure to natural light and the calming effects of nature can regulate sleep patterns.

• Increased Energy Levels: Forest bathing revitalizes the body and mind, providing a natural energy boost. It counteracts the fatigue and burnout often associated with urban living.

Parameters of Forest Bathing:

Forest bathing is a flexible practice that can be adapted to individual preferences and needs. However, some key parameters include:

• Mindful Presence: The practice emphasizes mindfulness, encouraging individuals to be fully present in the forest environment. This involves engaging all the senses—sight, sound, touch, taste, and smell.

• Slow Pacing: Forest bathing is not a hike or a race. It involves moving slowly, sometimes barely covering any distance at all. The focus is on the quality of the experience rather than quantity.

• Solo or Guided: Forest bathing can be done individually or with the guidance of a certified forest therapy guide who facilitates the experience, providing prompts and activities to enhance mindfulness.

• No Technology: Disconnecting from electronic devices is crucial during forest bathing. The aim is to unplug from the digital world and connect with the natural world.

• Seasonal Variation: Forest bathing can be enjoyed year-round, with each season offering a unique sensory experience. Participants can witness the changing colors of leaves, the blooming of flowers, or the tranquility of a snow-covered forest.

• Openness to Exploration: Forest bathing encourages curiosity and exploration. It invites participants to interact with the environment by touching trees, feeling the texture of leaves, or simply sitting and observing.

Conclusion:

Forest bathing is a practice that invites individuals to slow down, engage with nature, and reap the numerous physical and psychological benefits it offers. It is an opportunity to reconnect with our natural environment, reduce stress, and foster a sense of well-being in an increasingly fast-paced and urbanized world. Whether practiced alone or with a guide, forest bathing provides a sanctuary of tranquility where the healing power of nature can be fully appreciated and harnessed for holistic wellness.

Examples of Places Worldwide Utilizing Forest Bathing:

Forest bathing has gained popularity globally, and many locations worldwide offer forest bathing experiences. Here are a few notable examples:

Japan: Shinrin-yoku originated in Japan, and the country is home to numerous designated forest therapy trails and areas. The Yakushima Island and the Japanese Alps are well-known destinations for forest bathing.

South Korea: South Korea has embraced forest therapy as a form of relaxation and stress relief. The Healing Forest Center on Jeju Island is a prominent spot for forest bathing activities.

United States: Forest bathing has gained traction in the United States, particularly in areas with lush forests. Places like Muir Woods National Monument in California and the Great Smoky Mountains National Park in Tennessee offer guided forest bathing experiences.

Canada: Canada boasts vast forests, making it an ideal location for forest bathing. The Ancient Forest Alliance in British Columbia provides opportunities for this practice.

Scotland: The concept of "Shinrin-yoku" has been embraced in Scotland, where forest therapy guides lead sessions in serene natural settings like the Scottish Highlands.

Finland: Finnish Lapland offers forest bathing experiences, allowing visitors to connect with the Arctic wilderness and experience the calming effects of nature.

Australia: The Dandenong Ranges near Melbourne and the Tarkine Wilderness in Tasmania are among the Australian locations that offer forest bathing sessions.

Taiwan: Taiwan has embraced the concept of forest bathing with forest therapy trails in various national parks, including Alishan National Scenic Area and Yangmingshan National Park.

Norway: Norway's expansive forests and serene landscapes provide an excellent backdrop for forest bathing, with guided sessions available in various regions.

United Kingdom: The Forest of Dean in England and the Galloway Forest Park in Scotland offer opportunities for forest bathing, allowing participants to immerse themselves in the beauty of nature.

These are just a few examples of places worldwide that recognize the therapeutic benefits of forest bathing and offer guided experiences to help individuals connect with nature, reduce stress, and improve overall well-being. Forest bathing is a practice that encourages people to slow down, engage their senses, and find healing in the tranquility of forests.

What is also a great benefit is Community Healing Circles have facilitated gatherings where participants come together in a safe environment to share and discuss their personal experiences, traumas, or concerns to find collective understanding, support, healing, and sometimes even address broader community or social issues.

Historically, many indigenous and traditional societies around the world practiced some form of circle gathering for decision-making, conflict resolution, and communal healing. In addition to these traditional circles, the 60s and 70s saw the rise of encounter groups or support groups. These were sessions where individuals gathered, often without a therapist, to achieve personal change through intense and open emotional interactions. These groups emphasized:

Holistic Approach: Focusing on the emotional, spiritual, physical, and mental aspects of individuals.Equity: Everyone in the circle is treated as an equal, ensuring that every voice is heard.Sacred Rituals: Incorporating elements such as prayers, chants, or ceremonial practices.Restorative Justice: Rather than punitive measures, these circles often aimed to restore harmony in the community.

Examples Around the World:

Talking Circles (North America): Used by Native Americans, these are gatherings where participants speak one at a time, often using a talking stick. It's a way to discuss issues or concerns and ensure every voice is heard.

Peacemaking Circles (USA): Rooted in indigenous traditions, these circles are used in some U.S. communities for conflict resolution and restorative justice, particularly among youth.

Ubuntu Circles (South Africa): Derived from the philosophy of "Ubuntu" (I am because we are), these circles were instrumental during the Truth and Reconciliation Commission to address the traumas of apartheid.

Family Group Conferences (New Zealand): Rooted in Maori tradition, these are used in the child welfare and justice systems to make decisions involving a child.

Sentencing Circles (Canada): Used in some parts of Canada, particularly among indigenous communities, for restorative justice in the legal system.

Halaqa (Middle East): An Islamic tradition where people gather, often in a circle, to study and discuss religious texts and issues.

Council of Elders (Many Indigenous Cultures): In numerous societies, elders gather in circles to make decisions and provide guidance to their communities.

Encounter Groups (Global, particularly in the USA): Popularized in the 60s and 70s, these groups encouraged participants to openly express their emotions and confront issues in their lives, often in a setting without a traditional therapist. The goal was personal growth and understanding through intense emotional interactions.

In modern times, the concept of healing circles and support groups has been embraced and adapted by various groups and organizations to address a plethora of societal and communal issues, such as trauma from violence, substance abuse recovery, and building community resilience.

While the forms and names of these circles might differ, the core principle remains the same: creating a safe and inclusive space for open dialogue, mutual respect, and communal healing.

Conclusion

As we draw the narrative to a close, we reflect upon the profound depth of Zen-inspired healing practices and their transformative impact in contemporary healthcare settings. Through a rich mosaic of case studies and testimonials, we showcase the holistic and nurturing approach Zen principles foster, offering a path to healing that is deeply human and inclusive. This presentation, steeped in narratives of healing and recovery, invites viewers to envision a healthcare landscape that embraces the profound wisdom of Zen, fostering spaces of healing that are rooted in empathy, understanding, and deep respect for the intricate tapestry of the human experience, encouraging a harmonious balance and a nurturing spirit, celebrating the profound interconnectedness of all dimensions of the human experience. It leaves the audience with a hopeful vision of a future where healthcare is not just about curing ailments but nurturing the holistic well-being of every individual, championing a path of recovery that is compassionate, inclusive, and deeply nurturing. It evokes a future resonating with the sound of healing, a symphony of therapies that celebrate the spirit of resilience, joy, and the beautiful journey of becoming whole again.

Chapter 2: The Mindful Physician

In the realm of healthcare, mindfulness stands as a beacon of hope, promising a route to more compassionate and effective medical practice. It refers to the conscious endeavor to stay present, focusing on the here and now rather than being lost in the whirlpool of past regrets or future anxieties. A mindful physician leverages this principle to foster a deep understanding of the patients, attending to their needs with an open heart and an attentive mind.

In a medical setting, heightened awareness can be seen as a disciplined approach to focus on the current moment, and to be wholly present during patient interactions, diagnosis, and treatment planning. This implies not just a focused approach toward understanding the physical symptoms presented by the patients but extends to a conscious engagement with their emotional narratives, fears, and hopes, encouraging a healthcare pathway that is both empathetic and precise.

Understanding mindfulness demands delving deep into the principles of awareness, acceptance, and non-judgmental presence. It involves an active process of tuning into one's feelings and thoughts while also being equally receptive to the narratives of others. In a medical scenario, this translates to a practitioner's ability to keenly listen to the patient, empathize with their condition, and carve a healing path that respects the individuality of each patient. It stands as a tool that fosters a nurturing physician-patient relationship, where mutual respect and understanding are the cornerstones.

As a principle, enhanced wakefulness advocates for a kind of presence that is rooted in the now. In a healthcare setting, this means creating a space where patients can feel seen and heard, where their narratives are not just acknowledged but become a central part of the healing journey. This involves a compassionate approach to medical practice where the physician not just heals with medicines but also with words, understanding, and a nurturing presence that fosters a sense of trust and safety.

By fostering a mindful approach to medical practice, physicians embark on a journey that not just heals the body but also touches the soul, promising a healthcare pathway that is as compassionate as it is efficient, a journey marked with empathy, understanding, and a deep respect for the sanctity of human life and experiences. It evokes a vision of healthcare that is nurturing, that sees the individual not just as a patient but as a narrative of experiences, fears, and hopes, encouraging a healing path that is both humane and profoundly respectful of the individual journey that each patient traverses in their pathway to recovery.

Psychological Foundations of Enhancement Consciousness.

As we venture into the realm of understanding the psychological foundations of mindfulness, it is imperative to traverse the landscapes of consciousness, cognition, and emotional regulation, elements that stand central to this discourse. Here, we delve deep into the psychological tapestry that supports mindfulness, painting a picture that not only explains but also invites individuals to experience the richness that evolved awareness brings to the human psyche.

Understanding the psychological dynamics that govern mindfulness requires a comprehensive exploration of cognitive behavioral theories, neurobiology, and psychotherapy approaches, which converge to form the backbone of mindfulness practices. Through this lens, we unravel how mindfulness can be a potent tool in fostering mental well-being, enhancing attention, and reducing stress.

Understanding the psychological underpinnings of evolved, consciousness, takes us on a deep dive into the realms of cognitive science and human behavior. Here, the principles of neuroplasticity stand prominent, illustrating how consistent mindfulness practices can reshape our neural pathways, fostering a mind that is more resilient, adaptable, and attuned to the present moment.

Further, the cognitive behavioral approach to heightened consciousness highlights the role of meta-cognitive processes, where individuals learn to detach from automatic responses and foster a kind of awareness that is non-judgmental and rooted in the present. This not only promotes a greater sense of self-awareness but also a compassionate outlook towards oneself and others, facilitating a harmonious interaction with the world around us.

As we weave through the intricate layers of psychological foundations, we understand that mindfulness stands as a beacon in the chaotic modern world. It offers a path of tranquility, a journey of returning to oneself, of fostering an inner sanctuary of peace and stability, a refuge that encourages self-exploration and a harmonious existence with the outer world. It presents a pathway to healing, an avenue to rediscover the joy of being, and a nurturing embrace that holds the promise of a more conscious, compassionate, and mindful existence. It beckons individuals to step into a space of awareness where each moment is lived fully, where life unfolds in its rich tapestry of experiences, beckoning a deeper connection, understanding, and a profound celebration of the present moment.

As we delve into the nuanced landscapes of evolved consciousness, and its juxtaposition against related concepts, we unearth rich terrains of understanding, painting a vivid canvas of distinctions and interrelations that give rise to a more holistic comprehension. The inquiry takes us on a journey through various paradigms including, but not limited to, concentration, meditation, and cognitive behavioral therapy.

The journey to differentiate heightened awareness from related concepts invites us to delve deep into the core principles that govern this practice. At its core, mindfulness is rooted in the cultivation of moment-to-moment awareness, a conscious engagement with the present that stands distinct from mere concentration or focus.

In healthcare, mindfulness has emerged as a potent force, a tool that promises not only healing but a pathway to a more empathetic, compassionate, and conscious healthcare landscape. The role it carves is one of significant depth, fostering connections that go beyond the physical, venturing into the realms of emotional and psychological well-being

Defining the role of heightened awareness in healthcare invites us to explore a landscape rich with possibilities, where practitioners are encouraged to foster a deeper, more attuned connection with their patients. Here, mindfulness paves the way for a healthcare model rooted in empathy, where the holistic well-being of the patient stands central to the practice.

In this scenario, mindfulness stands as a beacon of hope, a tool that promises not only to heal but to foster a deeper connection, an engagement that is rooted in respect for the individual's holistic well-being. It paints a future of healthcare that is rooted in empathy, where the practitioner-patient relationship evolves into a nurturing ground of mutual respect and understanding, promising a pathway of healing that is both humane and profoundly respectful of the individual's health journey.

In the intricate pathways of healthcare, diagnostic accuracy stands as a pivotal aspect, a ground where the convergence of expertise and attention paves the way for successful outcomes. Here, mindfulness enters as a potent tool, promising to enhance the landscape of diagnostics, offering a pathway that is both precise and deeply attuned to the nuances of individual health narratives.

When we speak of mindfulness enhancing diagnostic accuracy, we refer to the ability of healthcare practitioners to be wholly present, fostering a keen awareness that encompasses not just the physical symptoms but a deep-seated understanding of the individual's holistic health landscape. It speaks of a cultivated presence that stands vigilant, keenly observing the subtle signs and narratives that often remain unheard, undiagnosed in the hurried pathways of modern healthcare.

Understanding this aspect takes us on a journey through the realms of diagnostic pathways where mindfulness promises to be a beacon of hope, encouraging practitioners to slow down, to engage with a keen sense of awareness that is open, receptive, and deeply connected to the individual narratives.

Here, the role of evoking consciousness extends to fostering a diagnostic pathway that is not just about identifying diseases but understanding the individual in a deeper context. It encourages a narrative where diagnostics is a dialogue, a space of understanding that fosters a deeper engagement with the patient, where the practitioner is encouraged to look beyond the obvious, venturing into a space of intuitive understanding, fostered through a deeply attuned presence.

In this space, mindfulness emerges as a potent tool in the diagnostic toolkit, a practice that fosters a keen awareness, a deep-seated engagement that promises to enhance the accuracy, precision, and depth of diagnostic pathways. It beckons a future where diagnostics is not just a technical endeavor but a conscious engagement, a dialogue fostered through presence, understanding, and a deep-seated respect for the sanctity of individual health narratives, promising a future of healthcare that is both precise and profoundly respectful of the individual journey that each patient traverses in their pathway to recovery.

Mindfulness Techniques for Physicians' Daily Practices

Understanding the principles of mindfulness and bringing them into daily routines can play a pivotal role in enhancing a physician's ability to focus, connect, and maintain well-being. These techniques aim to promote a more empathetic and compassionate approach to healthcare, bringing about a level of focus that is both rejuvenating and grounding.

To delve deeper, we look at the daily routines and habits that can foster mindfulness. It might involve beginning the day with mindfulness meditation, which grounds the physicians and helps them connect with their inner selves. They could engage in mindful walking, where attention is given to every step, promoting a moment of calm in a busy day. The incorporation of these techniques into daily routines nurtures a healthcare environment that emphasizes care, empathy, and complete presence.

Implementation could range from short, guided mindfulness exercises to help start the day on a focused note to utilizing mindful moments to reconnect with the present during a hectic day. These practices ensure continuity of care and empathy, enhancing the service provided to the patients while taking care of the physician.

At the core of stress reduction is mindful breathing, a practice that involves a deep focus on one's breath, facilitating a calming and grounding effect that aids in reducing stress and enhancing attention.

Physicians can be encouraged to take short breaks to focus on their breath, using it as a tool to bring them back to the present and reduce stress. These exercises can also be used in high-pressure situations to maintain calm and enhance focus, providing a grounding point in the chaotic environment of healthcare settings.

Heightened, focus, attention, in patient interaction, refers to being completely present during interactions, fostering an environment of trust and understanding through attentive listening and empathic responses.

This involves cultivating a practice of active listening, where the physician is present fully in the conversation, giving space to the patient to express themselves while responding with empathy and understanding. This approach fosters a sense of trust and mutual respect, enhancing the quality of the healthcare service provided.

Application involves structured training where physicians learn to interact mindfully, ensuring that they maintain eye contact, and actively listen to the patients, nurturing a relationship grounded in trust and mutual respect, and fostering a healing environment.

Here, the emphasis is on nurturing a positive and dynamic healthcare landscape where feedback is actively incorporated into the practice, fostering a nurturing environment grounded in respect and the desire to continually evolve and grow.

As we traverse the pathways of patient interaction, the role of mindfulness becomes even more significant. Being completely present during interactions fosters an environment of trust and understanding, enhancing the quality of healthcare services. Here, the cultivation of active listening skills stands as a crucial element, nurturing a relationship grounded in empathy and mutual respect.

Lastly, we touch upon the role of mindfulness in patient Inn reviews, a space where feedback becomes a tool for growth and improvement. By approaching reviews with an open heart and a willingness to grow, healthcare services can evolve dynamically, incorporating feedback to enhance the patient experience, and fostering an environment grounded in respect and the desire to offer a nurturing, patient-centric approach.

As we look towards a future of healthcare that is dynamically evolving, the role of mindfulness stands as a beacon of hope, promising a pathway grounded in empathy, mutual respect, and a conscious, present engagement, fostering an environment of healing and well-being.

In the context of healthcare, mindfulness in patient relationships refers to the practice of being fully present, attentive, and consciously engaging with patients to foster a nurturing, trusting, and understanding environment. This demands a proactive approach to fostering relationships grounded in empathy, active listening, and mutual respect.

To understand the depth of mindful and heightened compassioned patient relationships, we delve into various techniques such as active listening where physicians are encouraged to be fully present, immersing themselves in the narratives shared by the patients, to foster a genuine understanding. This approach extends beyond verbal communication to include non-verbal cues, fostering a deeper connection and understanding.

Utilizing mental and emotional presence in establishing patient relationships not only enhances communication but also cultivates a space where patients feel seen, heard, and understood. The practice encourages the incorporation of patience, kindness, and empathy, aiding in a richer understanding of the patient's experiences and concerns, thus building a substantial foundation for a trusting relationship.

Implementing heightened awareness, in patient relationships involves creating spaces for open communication where patients can share their experiences without fear of judgment. Techniques such as reflective listening, where physicians mirror back the feelings and sentiments expressed by the patients, can be instrumental in building rapport.

Furthermore, physicians can be trained to foster a nurturing attitude, where they approach each interaction with an open heart and a readiness to understand the diverse perspectives and experiences of the patients. Regular mindfulness meditation sessions can also be integrated into the daily routines of healthcare professionals, helping them to cultivate a mindful approach to patient interactions, being fully present, and responsive to the patients' needs and concerns.

Building trust and understanding in a healthcare setting involves a conscious effort to foster a safe, respectful, and empathetic environment where patients feel valued and understood, paving the way for more fruitful physician-patient relationships.

To nurture trust and understanding, healthcare providers are encouraged to approach each interaction with sincerity and respect, creating a space where patients can express themselves freely. This would mean giving patients the time they need to express themselves, acknowledging their feelings, and validating their experiences.

Techniques like open-ended questioning can foster a deeper understanding, encouraging patients to share more, while a non-judgmental approach ensures that trust is maintained. Moreover, understanding and respecting the cultural and personal backgrounds of the patients can greatly enhance trust and foster a more inclusive healthcare environment.

The pathway to a fruitful physician-patient relationship is grounded in the conscious cultivation of mindfulness, where each interaction is approached with empathy, understanding, and respect, nurturing a healthcare landscape that is receptive, inclusive, and profoundly rooted in the principles of heightened awareness, paving the way for enhanced healthcare outcomes grounded in trust and mutual respect. Through this practice, we foster a healthcare environment where patients feel valued and understood, enhancing not only the healthcare outcomes but also the holistic well-being of both the healthcare providers and the patients they serve.

The role of active listening cannot be understated in the process of enhancing diagnostic accuracy through mindfulness. Active listening involves more than just hearing the words a patient says; it includes understanding the emotions and intentions behind those words. This empathic approach to listening fosters a deeper understanding of the patient's concerns and can often uncover underlying issues that may be contributing to the patient's health condition.

Some concrete examples of institutions that are using Haydn's awareness and Zen principles as part of their outlook on patient care

Johns Hopkins Medicine in the USA is one of the pioneers in implementing mindfulness-based stress reduction (MBSR) programs, catering not just to patients but also to healthcare providers. This holistic approach has registered a decrease in burnout levels among healthcare providers and improved patient satisfaction through more attentive and empathic care. The initiative brought to light that regular mindfulness training could indeed be a cornerstone in enhancing the mental well-being of both the patients and the healthcare providers, fostering a nurturing and supportive environment.

The University of Massachusetts Medical School, through its established Center for Mindfulness in Medicine, Health Care, and Society, has been conducting MBSR programs, leading to remarkable improvements in the patient-doctor relationship and clinical outcomes. The center underscores that structured mindfulness training can indeed foster a healthcare environment where patients feel more satisfied, and clinical outcomes are optimized, highlighting the immense potential of adopting a formal approach to mindfulness training in healthcare settings.

Across the pond, the NHS in the UK has integrated mindfulness training in various trusts to help manage work-related stress and augment the quality of patient care. The results have been encouraging, illustrating a dip in staff turnover rates, improved mental well-being of healthcare providers, and enriched patient-provider relationships. This initiative highlights that mindfulness training is not just about individual well-being, but it transforms the work environment into a healthy space while sustaining a high-quality healthcare delivery system.

The benefits reaped from such initiatives are manifold. Mindfulness practices in healthcare facilitate a nurturing environment that takes into account the mental well-being of both patients and healthcare providers, creating a healthcare setting that promotes diagnostic accuracy and enhances patient outcomes.

The cultivation and nurturing of active listening skills through mindfulness programs have also been a notable outcome. Such skills foster a deeper and more empathic patient-doctor relationship, which has proven to lead to more accurate diagnoses. This approach not only ensures that healthcare providers are tuned into the verbal cues but also the non-verbal cues, offering a richer understanding of the patient's condition.

Conclusion

In wrapping up, the role of mindfulness in enhancing diagnostic accuracy presents a multifaceted approach to healthcare that is both compassionate and precise. When healthcare practitioners foster a habit of being fully present and attentive, they pave the way for a diagnostic process that is receptive and finely tuned to the individual narratives of each patient. Through a conscientious engagement grounded in mindfulness, physicians can significantly enhance the accuracy and reliability of their diagnostics, promising a healthcare pathway that respects and honors the intricate tapestry of individual health narratives, leading to a more patient-centered and effective approach to healthcare.

These case studies underline a substantial positive shift in the medical landscape brought about by the integration of heightened awareness into medical practice. Healthcare institutions around the world are beginning to recognize and reap the rewards of fostering this principle in their day-to-day operations. These case studies portray a future medical landscape steeped in attentiveness, empathy, and a focused approach, promising a healthcare ecosystem that is harmonious and tuned to the holistic well-being of all individuals involved. The road ahead looks promising, steering the healthcare sector toward an environment where mindfulness is not just an add-on but an essential fabric of healthcare delivery. It fosters a medical landscape that stands on a foundation of empathy and respect, promising better outcomes for all.

In the intricate healthcare ecosystem, mindful self-care for physicians stands as a pillar that upholds the structure of quality healthcare. The role of mindfulness in fostering self-care has been brought to the forefront with successful implementations in leading healthcare institutions globally. Delving deeper, we find that these self-care routines comprise not just meditation sessions, but also workshops that foster a community of shared experiences and support. Here, physicians learn to navigate the pressures of their demanding roles, leaning on mindfulness as a guide to balance and harmony. They are equipped with tools to handle stressful situations with calm and composure, nurturing a resilient mindset that aids in warding off the symptoms of burnout before they escalate.

As we broaden our understanding of the role of mindfulness in avoiding burnout, we find that it's a multi-pronged strategy involving individual and organizational efforts. Individuals learn to nurture a sense of self-compassion, giving themselves the grace to step back when needed and recharge. Institutions play a supportive role, facilitating environments that prioritize the mental well-being of their staff, often incorporating quiet rooms for meditation and reflection, encouraging regular breaks, and fostering open communication where concerns can be aired without fear of retribution. The initiative taken by the NHS in the UK stands as a testament to the potential success of such approaches, with their mindfulness training not only helping in averting burnout but also enhancing the work satisfaction and efficiency of their staff.

The early recognition of the signs of burnout is yet another critical facet of this discourse. Mindfulness, with its emphasis on being present and fully engaged with the current scenario, facilitates a heightened awareness of one's mental and physical state. Healthcare providers learn to tune into their bodies, recognizing early symptoms like persistent fatigue, disillusionment, and a detached demeanor toward their duties. Training in focused, meditation equips them with the ability to perceive these signs in a non-judgmental manner, creating a space for early interventions that could include seeking support, adjusting workloads, or taking necessary breaks to replenish their energy. The fostering of such self-awareness has been a hallmark of the programs implemented at centers such as the University of Massachul

It is evident from the diverse range of case studies that mindfulness serves as an effective antidote to the pressing issue of burnout in the healthcare sector. It nurtures a culture where the well-being of healthcare providers is given paramount importance, understanding that a caregiver in the optimum state of mind and health can offer the best care to patients.

Within the vast spectrum of healthcare delivery, building a resilient self emerges as a proactive measure that protects healthcare professionals from the burnout that comes from the high-stress environment in which they operate. The question then arises, how can one foster resilience through mindfulness?

The foundational stages involve inculcating mindfulness practices that enhance self-awareness, a pivotal step toward resilience. The teachings from renowned institutions such as Johns Hopkins Medicine and the University of Massachusetts Medical School have fostered mindfulness interventions, encouraging healthcare professionals to cultivate a habit of regular self-check-ins. These check-ins involve a conscious pausing to assess one's mental and emotional state, allowing for a timely identification of stressors and addressing them promptly before they escalate.

Moreover, building resilience through mindfulness entails developing a robust personal practice where the core principles of mindfulness, such as present-moment awareness and non-judgmental acknowledgment of experiences, are internalized. It might involve structured training sessions where healthcare providers are taught to approach challenges with a balanced perspective, not getting swayed by the highs and lows but maintaining a steady, centered approach.

An essential aspect of fostering resilience is learning to cultivate self-compassion, a lesson deeply ingrained in mindfulness teachings. Healthcare providers are encouraged to extend the same compassion they offer to their patients themselves, recognizing when they need to step back, rest, and rejuvenate. It is through nurturing self-compassion that they can prevent burnout and maintain a sustainable, long-term commitment to their profession.

Turning towards more practical realms, healthcare institutions have started implementing peer support groups facilitated by mindfulness experts. These groups serve as safe havens where experiences are shared, and collective mindfulness exercises are undertaken to build community resilience. The underlying philosophy is fostering a sense of belonging and understanding, leveraging the collective energy to build individual resilience.

In conclusion, building a resilient self through mindfulness is a multifaceted approach, involving individual and community efforts guided by expert interventions. Through systematic integration of mindfulness practices into the healthcare ecosystem, there emerges a ripple effect where personal resilience builds a robust and resilient workforce, effectively improving the healthcare delivery system.

The lesson drawn from various case studies urges healthcare settings globally to adopt a resilience-focused approach, nurturing healthcare professionals who are not just skilled but resilient warriors, equipped to navigate the complexities of their profession with grace, balance, and strength. It paints a vision of a healthcare landscape where resilience is not just a buzzword but a lived reality, fostered through mindfulness practices deeply entrenched in the daily workings of healthcare systems, paving the path for a healthier, harmonious, and more effective healthcare delivery system.

Chapter 3: Compassionate Care

As we delve into chapter 3, we address the profound role of compassionate care in healthcare settings, leveraging the rich learning from mindfulness principles to elucidate the science of compassion, its psychological perspectives, and the neurological basis grounding it.

The science of compassion finds its foundations in our very biology. From a biological viewpoint, compassion is seen as a natural and automatic response that has evolved to facilitate cooperation and protection of the group. It involves a complex interplay of various hormonal and neural networks, working cohesively to foster a sense of empathy and understanding towards others. Delving into mindfulness teachings, we find that the cultivation of compassion is fundamentally intertwined with the practice of being present and fully immersing oneself in the experiences of others, a gesture that not only fosters deeper connections but also facilitates healing and well-being.

From a psychological perspective, compassion extends beyond mere understanding; it involves actively wishing to relieve the suffering of others. Psychologists propound that compassion is an offshoot of empathy, yet it goes a step further by involving a genuine desire to help. Mindfulness practices foster this depth of understanding and responsiveness, nurturing a mental space where healthcare providers are not just listeners but are actively engaged in alleviating distress, employing not just their expertise but their deep-seated empathy and compassionate disposition to offer care that heals both physically and emotionally.

Understanding the knowledge neurological basis of compassion brings us to a fascinating intersection of mindfulness and neuroscience. Recent studies have begun to uncover the neural pathways and brain regions involved in compassion. The anterior insula and anterior cingulate cortex, for instance, play pivotal roles in empathic responses, generating a visceral understanding of another person's experience.

Moreover, mindfulness practices, as advocated in various healthcare setups globally, facilitate the strengthening of these neural pathways, fostering a brain that is more attuned to compassionate responses.

Moreover, the practice of focused meditation has been seen to enhance activity in regions of the brain associated with emotional regulation and positive emotions, thereby fostering a heightened sense of compassion. Through regular mindfulness exercises that emphasize compassionate thinking, healthcare professionals can essentially 'train their brain' to respond with more compassion, enhancing their ability to connect with their patients on a deeper level and offering care that is truly empathetic.

Furthermore, it is crucial to foster an environment where healthcare professionals can practice self-compassion, understanding and forgiving themselves, a practice that is grounded in the principles of mindfulness. This nurturing of self-compassion forms a basis from which outward compassion flows, facilitating a healthcare environment that is understanding, patient, and genuinely caring.

In conclusion, compassionate care stands as a beacon of hope, a practice that aligns beautifully with the mindfulness principles fostering a healthcare system that is grounded in science yet enriched with deep compassion, understanding, and empathy. Through a deep understanding of the neurological underpinnings and psychological perspectives on compassion, healthcare setups globally are positioned to foster a nurturing environment, where compassionate care is not just a practice but a culture, embodying a holistic approach to healthcare that is grounded in science yet elevated with genuine care and empathy.

Understanding the Neurological Basis of Compassion

At the outset, to unravel the neurological basis of compassion, one must turn attention towards the brain's intricate mechanism that facilitates empathic engagements. Neuroscience has enabled us to comprehend that several brain regions, including the anterior cingulate cortex and the anterior insula, are pivotal in driving compassion, a process intricately linked with the perception of others' pain and the ensuing empathic concern that leads to a desire to alleviate that suffering.

The role of mirror neurons is equally crucial in this context, facilitating a mechanism where we almost vicariously experience others' emotions, fostering a profound understanding and a nurturing ground for compassion to flourish. Through mindfulness practices, individuals can potentially enhance the functionality of these neurological pathways, enriching the depth of compassion one can extend to others.

When we traverse the pathway delineating compassion from sympathy, it is imperative to highlight that while both stem from a place of understanding and concern, they differ significantly in their depth and engagement levels. Sympathy often involves a feeling of pity or sorrow for someone else's misfortune, generally from a distant perspective.

On the other hand, compassion delves much deeper, encouraging a more engaged and active involvement in understanding and alleviating the other person's suffering. It entails not only recognizing the suffering but immersing oneself in the emotional landscape of the individual, fostering a genuine desire to alleviate the distress. Through mindfulness practices, healthcare professionals can cultivate a genuine approach towards compassion, building connections that are deeply rooted in understanding, empathy, and a firm desire to foster healing and well-being.

As we advance to delineate compassion from healing, it becomes clear that while the two concepts are deeply intertwined, they represent different facets of the caregiving process. Compassion forms the bedrock of the healing process, steering it with empathy and deep understanding, guiding the approach to patient care with sensitivity and humane touch.

However, healing extends beyond the realm of emotional engagement to include a comprehensive process involving medical interventions, therapeutic processes, and recuperative care to restore an individual's health. Healing is a more encompassing term representing a journey towards recovery, potentially driven and facilitated by compassionate care.

Heightened consciousness,, in this context, stands as a potent tool that bridges compassion and healing, encouraging healthcare professionals to approach the healing process with a compassionate lens. It fosters a realm where healing is not just about physical recovery but encompasses a holistic approach that considers the emotional, psychological, and spiritual well-being of the individuals.

Through a more detailed exploration of the neurological pathways fostering compassion, and understanding the nuanced differences between compassion, sympathy, and healing, we stand at a juncture where healthcare can truly transcend from being a mere provision of medical services to a deeply humane process guided by understanding, empathy, and a profound desire to foster well-being in its truest sense.

By employing enhanced, focusing practices, healthcare professionals can steer the trajectory of healthcare to a landscape that is deeply nurturing, establishing a harmonious bridge between science and the human touch, between medical interventions and heartfelt compassion, crafting a healthcare narrative that is not only effective but deeply nurturing, kind, and profoundly compassionate.

However, excessive empathy often puts individuals at risk of emotional burnout, a state characterized by emotional exhaustion and a decrease in personal accomplishment. Constantly absorbing others' feelings and perspectives can become extremely draining over time.

This is heightened in high-pressure environments, such as healthcare, where professionals are constantly bearing witness to a spectrum of human suffering and distress. It could potentially affect one's mental health negatively, spiraling into a state of chronic fatigue where one finds it hard to find joy and fulfillment in their role. Developing coping strategies such as engaging in regular physical activity, pursuing a hobby, or seeking therapy could be vital in mitigating the effects of emotional burnout.

Individuals with excessive empathy may struggle to establish and maintain personal and professional boundaries. This can lead to a loss of self, as they continuously prioritize others' needs over their own. The difficulty in delineating the self from others can further lead to confusion, stress, and feeling overwhelmed. In healthcare settings, it becomes even more imperative to have clearly defined boundaries to avoid getting too emotionally entangled with patients, which might impair the professional's ability to make impartial decisions. By honing skills like assertiveness and learning to say no, individuals can foster healthier relationships and protect their own emotional well-being.

The dilemma of being extremely empathic often involves a blurred line between being understanding and losing oneself in others' experiences, which can cause decision-making challenges. In a healthcare scenario, it can potentially compromise the quality of service as professionals might become overly involved, overlooking critical information that demands a rational approach. It is essential to find a harmonious balance where one can empathize with others without losing sight of the larger picture that includes well-informed, rational decision-making based on facts and not solely on emotions.

Mastering the art of navigating complex emotional landscapes entails a deeper understanding of oneself and others. It is a continual process where one learns to differentiate between their emotions and the emotions of others. This self-awareness could be fostered through consistent self-reflection and possibly, Zen meditation. In healthcare, professionals would benefit from training that helps in identifying and managing their emotional responses adequately, enhancing their ability to provide compassionate care without feeling overwhelmed.

Practicing heightened awareness and engaging in self-reflection are potent tools in navigating emotional terrains effectively. Mindfulness aids individuals in staying grounded, creating a buffer against the onslaught of external emotional stimuli. In healthcare settings, embedding mindfulness into the daily routine can offer a sanctuary of calm, enabling professionals to revisit their inner equilibrium, thus nurturing their mental health. Reflective practices also offer avenues for personal growth, facilitating a deeper understanding of oneself and the dynamics of interpersonal relationships.

Communication goes beyond verbal expression; it involves non-verbal cues, active listening, and a genuine understanding of the other person's standpoint. Developing refined communication skills is akin to crafting a bridge that facilitates smoother interpersonal interactions. For healthcare professionals, honing these skills could translate to establishing a trusting and respectful relationship with patients, thereby enhancing the healing environment and potentially improving the outcome of the treatments.

Emotional intelligence is pivotal in fostering patient-centered care. It enables healthcare providers to resonate with their patients, to tune into their frequencies and comprehend their fears, anxieties, and expectations. This level of understanding allows for a more individualized approach to care, nurturing a therapeutic alliance with patients. Moreover, it aids in anticipating the needs of the patients, sometimes even before they voice them, thereby fostering an environment of trust and mutual respect.

In a healthcare setting, the dynamics between team members significantly influence the work environment and, by extension, the quality of care provided to patients. A high level of emotional intelligence promotes a culture of understanding, cooperation, and collaboration, fostering a harmonious work environment. It involves being tuned to one's own emotions as well as being sensitive to the emotional cues of colleagues, which paves the way for constructive feedback and collaborative problem-solving.

Healthcare settings can be extremely demanding, requiring professionals to manage their stress levels adequately to avoid burnout. Emotional intelligence aids in recognizing early signs of stress and adopting strategies to counteract it effectively. Incorporating relaxation techniques, finding support systems, and seeking avenues for recreation can be critical in maintaining a healthy work-life balance. Moreover, emotional intelligence empowers individuals to seek help when needed, without succumbing to the pressures of the environment.

Healthcare professionals often find themselves at crossroads where they encounter ethical dilemmas. Navigating these complex situations requires a nuanced understanding of human emotions and ethical principles. Emotional intelligence aids in grasping the intricacies of these dilemmas, offering a perspective that is both compassionate and grounded in moral principles. It facilitates communication that is sensitive yet firm, helping in articulating difficult decisions while maintaining a semblance of empathy and understanding. Moreover, it helps in building a reservoir of resilience, aiding professionals in bouncing back after facing morally distressing situations.

Developing skills to navigate intricate emotional terrains is paramount in personal and professional life. This process begins with an individual fostering a deep understanding of their emotional responses and triggers. In environments characterized by high emotional volatility, it becomes vital to distinguish one's emotions from the collective emotional experience. It means cultivating an acute awareness of the emotional undercurrents in various situations and learning to respond rather than react. Developing such skills would involve educating oneself on psychological concepts, possibly attending workshops and therapy to get a grounded understanding of emotional dynamics.

Mindfulness and reflection become critical tools in one's arsenal when navigating complex emotional landscapes. The essence of mindfulness is to be present in the moment, a practice that allows for a heightened awareness of one's emotional state without being swept away by it. Practices, such as meditation and conscious breathing, can equip individuals to stay grounded amidst emotional turmoil. Reflection, facilitates deeper understanding and learning from past experiences, thereby aiding in crafting more informed responses in future encounters. Encouraging a culture of reflection can help in personal growth and in building emotionally intelligent communities.

To navigate complex emotional landscapes effectively, one needs to foster excellent communication skills. These skills involve being an attentive listener, reading between the lines, and being sensitive to non-verbal cues. It goes beyond mere verbal exchanges and delves into the realm of understanding the emotions behind the words. In the context of relationships, be it personal or professional, nuanced communication skills can often be the bedrock of trust and mutual respect. Hence, honing communication skills becomes a vital component in navigating emotional landscapes adeptly.

To provide a very clear understanding

of empathy let us consider the following

Empathy is the ability to understand and share the feelings of another, placing oneself in their position emotionally and cognitively. And some of the pitfalls to avoid are as follows.

Emotional Exhaustion: Continually absorbing others' emotions can lead to burnout.Safeguard: Set boundaries. Learn to recognize when you're taking on too much and give yourself permission to step back.

Difficulty Differentiating Emotions: It might become challenging to distinguish between your feelings and those of others.Safeguard:

Practice self-awareness. Regularly check in with yourself to identify and label your emotions.

Relationship Strain: Over-empathizing can sometimes make you prioritize others' needs over your own.Safeguard: Establish clear boundaries in relationships and communicate them openly.

Neglecting Self-Care: Being overly attuned to others might make you neglect your well-being.Safeguard: Schedule regular self-care activities, like meditation, reading, or any activity you love.

Feeling Overwhelmed: Constantly feeling others' pain can be overwhelming.Safeguard: Limit exposure to negative or emotionally draining situations when possible.

Physical Symptoms: Over-empathy can manifest as physical ailments like headaches or fatigue.Safeguard: Ensure you're prioritizing sleep, nutrition, and physical activity.

Diminished Objectivity: Being too empathetic can cloud judgment, making it hard to see situations clearly.Safeguard: Seek outside perspectives. Talk to trusted friends or a therapist to get a more objective viewpoint.

To navigate the challenges of being empathic, it's crucial to find balance. Embrace the gift of empathy while also ensuring you prioritize your well-being.

Emotional Intelligence in Healthcare Settings

Patient-Centered Care

The healthcare environment is a collaborative space where team dynamics play a pivotal role in the efficacy of the service provided. Emotional intelligence fosters an atmosphere of mutual respect and understanding among team members. Being sensitive to the emotional currents flowing through the team and having the ability to respond with empathy and understanding can build a cohesive unit that works harmoniously. It encourages open communication, shared decision-making, and a supportive work culture where individuals feel valued and respected, which, in turn, translates to enhanced care for patients.

Working in healthcare settings comes with its share of stresses and pressures. The ability to manage one's emotional responses effectively, to remain calm under pressure, and to find ways to recharge is crucial in this environment. Emotional intelligence guides individuals in identifying signs of stress early on and enables them to employ strategies to maintain emotional equilibrium. Encouraging a culture that supports emotional well-being, through avenues such as regular debriefings and providing support systems, can be instrumental in mitigating stress and preventing burnout.

Healthcare settings often present professionals with ethical dilemmas that demand a careful and sensitive approach. Navigating these situations with a high degree of emotional intelligence allows for decisions that are both ethical and compassionate. Understanding the emotional nuances and the potential impact of decisions on all involved parties is vital. Developing skills to communicate tough decisions with empathy and respect, while staying grounded in ethical principles, can aid in maintaining trust and fostering a culture of moral resilience in healthcare settings. It involves nurturing a moral compass that is sensitive to the emotional landscapes of others while adhering to the foundational ethical principles guiding healthcare practice.

Engaging in Altruistic Actions

Zen emphasizes selfless service and encourages individuals to engage in altruistic actions, without expecting anything in return. Volunteering, helping others in times of need, and simple acts of kindness can be ways to cultivate compassion. Engaging in altruistic actions creates a cycle of positive energy, fostering compassion both in the individual and in the community.

While extending compassion to others, it is equally important to nurture self-compassion. Zen teaches the importance of being kind and understanding towards oneself, recognizing that everyone is on a learning journey. By fostering self-compassion, one creates a well of empathy and understanding from which they can extend compassion to others.

Ultimately, the cultivation of compassion through Zen involves integrating compassionate attitudes and behaviors into daily life. It is about embodying compassion in every action, word, and thought, thereby fostering a life that is deeply connected with others, characterized by understanding, empathy, and love. It might involve creating routines and practices that nurture a compassionate heart, such as daily meditations, reflective writing, and consciously practicing kindness in daily interactions.

Through a continuous practice and integration of Zen principles and meditation techniques, individuals can nurture a deep-seated compassion, not just as a trait but as a way of being, guiding their interactions and relationships with understanding and love. It is a journey of cultivating a heart that resonates with others, fostering connections that are deep, meaningful, and grounded in the principles of compassion and empathy.

The philosophical grounding of Zen, deeply rooted in the principles of interconnectedness and impermanence, serves as a rich soil for cultivating compassion. The teachings encourage an understanding of the deep connection that exists between all beings, thereby fostering a natural inclination towards compassion. Engaging deeply with these teachings through study and contemplation can offer insights into the nature of suffering and the role of compassion in alleviating it.

Literature across ages has echoed the tenets of compassion, emphasizing empathy, understanding, and kindness towards others. Many literary works, both fictional and non-fictional, offer rich insights into the human condition, encouraging readers to cultivate a compassionate stance towards others. Delving deep into literary explorations of compassion can provide a nuanced understanding of its significance in human society.

In the world of literature, compassion often plays a pivotal role in character development. Characters displaying a deep sense of compassion often resonate well with readers, serving as models for compassionate living. Analyzing characters through the lens of compassion in literary discussions can foster a deeper understanding of the role of empathy and understanding in human interactions.

In in medical teaching, universities and institutions, , the incorporation of teachings on compassion can be a transformative force, nurturing a generation of individuals grounded in empathy and understanding. Through the study of literature and philosophical texts that emphasize compassion, students can be encouraged to cultivate a compassionate outlook on life. This could involve critical discussions on literary works focused on compassion, encouraging students to reflect on the role of compassion in their lives.

Literature and teachings on compassion often provide practical guidance on cultivating a compassionate stance in real-life scenarios. They offer strategies and insights that can be incorporated into daily life, encouraging individuals to practice compassion actively. Creating platforms for discussing and reflecting on these teachings can foster a community where compassion is not just a concept but a lived reality.

Implementing a curriculum that intertwines compassion with literature and philosophical teachings can foster an environment where individuals are not only intellectually stimulated but are also guided towards a path of compassionate living. It can be a potent force, steering individuals towards a deeper understanding and practice of compassion, enriched by the depth of insights derived from literature and philosophical teachings on compassion.

As previously noted, practices in Zen, including Zazen and Kinhin, provide avenues for individuals to cultivate a compassionate heart. Through consistent practice, individuals learn to relate to others from a place of understanding and empathy, fostering relationships grounded in compassion. Encouraging the adoption of these mindful practices in daily routines can be a significant step towards nurturing compassion in communities.

Historically, literature has served as a rich repository of compassionate narratives, documenting the human capacity for understanding, empathy, and compassion through various epochs. Analyzing historical texts and narratives through a compassionate lens can offer profound insights into the evolving understanding of compassion in human society.

In the literary cosmos, compassionate characters often play a central role, illustrating the transformative power of compassion in human interactions. Creating critical discussions around the representation of compassion in literature can foster deeper understanding and might inspire individuals to cultivate a compassionate outlook in real life.

Integrating the theme of compassion into educational settings through the exploration of literary texts can foster a nurturing environment. By encouraging students to analyze and discuss the role of compassion in literary narratives, educators can stimulate a compassionate understanding, encouraging individuals to apply these principles in their daily interactions.

The teachings on compassion often offer a wealth of strategies and principles that individuals can apply in their daily lives. Creating platforms that encourage dialogue and reflection on these teachings can nurture a living practice of compassion, with individuals embodying the principles of empathy and understanding in their daily interactions.

Developing educational resources grounded in the rich teachings on compassion can be a transformative initiative. Through books, workshops, and interactive sessions that delve into the depths of compassionate teachings, communities can foster a culture grounded in empathy and understanding.

In conclusion, compassion stands as a pivotal concept in Zen, literature, and various teachings, offering a guiding philosophy for fostering understanding and empathy in society. By nurturing a deeper understanding through the exploration of Zen practices, literary narratives, and educational teachings on compassion, individuals and communities can embark on a path of compassionate living, characterized by empathy, understanding, and mutual respect. This endeavor involves both individual and communal efforts, with a focus on educational initiatives and practical applications of compassion in daily life.

Real-World Applications of Zen Teachings on Compassion

Zen teachings underscore the importance of compassionate listening, encouraging individuals to be fully present and attentive while interacting with others. This practice can be fostered in personal and professional environments, facilitating a space where individuals feel heard and valued. By adopting compassionate listening in real-world settings, individuals can build relationships grounded in mutual respect and understanding

Applying the Zen principle of self-compassion in real-world scenarios involves nurturing a kind and understanding attitude towards oneself. Individuals can learn to treat themselves with the same empathy and understanding they extend to others, fostering personal well-being and mental health. This principle can be applied in various settings including educational institutions, workplaces, and homes, promoting a culture of understanding and empathy.

All the world is a stage.

Zen encourages altruistic actions, prompting individuals to serve others selflessly. In the real world, this can translate to community-building initiatives rooted in compassion, where individuals come together to support each other without expecting anything in return. This approach fosters a positive and supportive community environment, where compassion is the guiding principle.

An integral component of the training should focus on mindfulness practices, equipping healthcare professionals with the skills to remain present and fully attuned to the patients' needs. The training can encompass strategies to foster mindful communication, which can enhance the quality of interactions with patients, promoting a caring and understanding healthcare environment.

Given the high-stress nature of healthcare settings, introducing healthcare professionals to meditative techniques can be a vital part of the training. Through guided meditation sessions, professionals can learn to manage stress more effectively, promoting a sense of calm and centeredness that can be a crucial asset in their demanding roles.

Workshops should incorporate training modules that emphasize the role of active listening and empathetic communication in patient care. Through interactive sessions and role-playing exercises, healthcare professionals can develop the skill of listening with a compassionate heart, facilitating a trust-rich environment that is conducive to healing.

Recognizing the strenuous nature of healthcare roles, the training should foster self-compassion among healthcare professionals. Workshops can introduce exercises and reflective practices that encourage professionals to treat themselves with kindness and understanding, helping to prevent burnout and sustain a long, fulfilling career in healthcare.

To foster a broader culture of compassion, training workshops should also address the role of community engagement. Through discussions and brainstorming sessions, professionals can explore opportunities for compassionate initiatives and outreach programs that serve to enhance the well-being of the community at large, encouraging a healthcare system that extends beyond the walls of medical facilities.

In conclusion, compassion training workshops stand as a beacon of hope in revolutionizing healthcare settings, fostering an environment grounded in empathy, understanding, and mutual respect. By integrating a rich array of strategies ranging from mindfulness practices to community engagement initiatives, these workshops aim to nurture a cadre of healthcare professionals equipped with the knowledge and skills to offer compassionate care. This approach not only transforms the patient-care provider relationship but also instills a deep-seated culture of compassion, paving the way for a healthcare system characterized by holistic well-being and nurturing care. Through sustained efforts in training and development, the goal is to cultivate a healthcare landscape that is synonymous with compassion, enhancing the quality of care and elevating the healthcare experience for all involved.

Implementing Zen Compassion Practices in Daily Routines for Both Practitioner and Patient

To initiate the incorporation of Zen compassion practices in daily routines, it is vital that both practitioners and patients first immerse themselves in understanding the fundamental principles of compassion. This entails recognizing the interconnectedness of all beings and nurturing a genuine desire to alleviate suffering. Establishing an understanding of these core principles sets a foundation for compassionate interactions in healthcare settings.

As part of the daily healthcare routine, integrating mindfulness can play a pivotal role. Practitioners and patients can be trained to maintain a state of present awareness, encouraging attentive and understanding interactions. Meditation techniques derived from Zen teachings could aid in developing a focused and attentive mind, enhancing the quality of healthcare experiences.

Incorporating Zen meditation sessions as a part of daily routines can assist in reducing stress and fostering a tranquil mindset for both practitioners and patients. This practice, grounded in Zen philosophies, aims to cultivate a space of inner peace, thereby facilitating a harmonious healthcare environment where both parties can engage with a calm and centered disposition.

An essential facet of Zen compassion practices involves fostering self-compassion. Workshops guiding both practitioners and patients in nurturing a compassionate stance towards oneself can be a transformative inclusion in daily routines. This approach encourages individuals to treat themselves with the same understanding and kindness they extend to others, promoting a sense of well-being and balance.

Zen teachings advocate for altruism and community building. In the healthcare setting, this can translate into initiatives where practitioners and patients alike engage in community-building endeavors, championing mutual support and understanding. This creates a nurturing environment where compassionate actions are at the forefront, encouraging a healthcare system that is both inclusive and empathetic.

The integration of Zen compassion practices in daily routines heralds a significant transformation in healthcare dynamics. By fostering understanding through the teachings of Zen, it sets a course for healthcare experiences that are deeply grounded in compassion, mindfulness, and empathetic engagement. Both practitioners and patients stand to benefit immensely from this compassionate approach, navigating the healthcare landscape with a sense of calm, understanding, and mutual respect. This initiative, grounded in the timeless wisdom of Zen teachings, envisions a healthcare sector that is synonymous with compassion and holistic well-being, nurturing a space of healing and understanding for all involved.

Case Studies: Compassionate Care in Action Supplying Success Stories and Narratives Showcasing the Positive Outcomes of Compassionate Care

In the landscape of healthcare, a deep understanding and implementation of the core principles of compassion have shown to foster a nurturing environment where both patients and practitioners thrive. Detailed case studies help in illustrating the successful implementation and the positive repercussions of basing healthcare on the principles of understanding, empathy, and a genuine desire to alleviate suffering.

Delving into real-life scenarios where mindfulness practices were applied showcases a marked enhancement in the quality of care and patient satisfaction. Narratives highlight how practitioners, grounded in the present moment, could understand the nuanced needs of the patients, paving the way for a healthcare experience that is both attentive and considerate.

In high-pressure environments such as emergency settings, the role of empathic communication becomes magnified. Case studies depict scenarios where open channels of understanding and empathetic communication have facilitated quicker responses and fostered a supportive environment, ultimately playing a crucial role in safeguarding the well-being of patients in crisis situations.

Within the strenuous environments of emergency settings, self-compassion initiatives take a center stage in several case studies. These narratives bring to light instances where practitioners who practiced self-compassion were able to recover faster and maintain a high level of care, even in back-to-back emergency situations, showcasing the sustaining power of self-kindness in crisis scenarios.

Community response and cohesion often become the bedrock of crisis management. Case studies unfold stories where communities came together, guided by the principles of compassionate care, aiding in efficient and heart-centered responses to emergencies. These stories highlight the unity and strength derived from compassionate community actions during crisis situations.

The range of case studies brings forward a rich narrative highlighting the vital role of compassion in emergency settings. Each case reflects the power of staying grounded in compassion and understanding even in the face of crisis, showcasing the remarkable outcomes when the principles of compassionate care are implemented in emergency settings. Through the lens of real-life scenarios, we witness the resilience, efficiency, and humanity that shines through when compassion becomes the guiding force in crisis situations. These cases stand as a testament to the profound impact compassionate care can impart, offering a beacon of hope and a pathway to more empathic, responsive, and successful outcomes in emergency healthcare settings.

Being mindful can be a strong ally in detecting the early signs of compassion fatigue. This segment would explore techniques such as self-monitoring and awareness practices to promptly identify signs of emotional exhaustion. Additionally, it would spotlight mindfulness approaches to remain vigilant towards signs of compassion fatigue in others, promoting a proactive approach to well-being

Leveraging meditation as a preventive measure against compassion fatigue holds immense potential. This section would introduce various meditation techniques aimed at nurturing resilience and maintaining emotional stability, effectively acting as a buffer against the onset of compassion fatigue.

Often, compassion fatigue leads to a sense of isolation. Here we would address the role of empathic communication in fostering connections and preventing isolation, which is a prominent sign of compassion fatigue. Techniques discussed would involve nurturing open dialogues and encouraging sharing of experiences to foster a supportive environment.

Creating robust support systems through community building emerges as a viable strategy in warding off compassion fatigue. This section would discuss collaborative efforts and peer support groups which can act as a safety net, offering support and understanding, and thereby playing a crucial role in preventing compassion fatigue.

Achieving a harmonious balance between compassion and self-care is a nuanced endeavor, requiring a grounded understanding in the core principles of compassion, coupled with advanced mindfulness and meditation practices, empathic communication skills, and a strong foundation in self-compassion. Through this detailed guide, individuals can navigate the intricacies of maintaining this balance, leveraging a rich set of tools and strategies that foster a harmonious, respectful, and nurturing environment both for oneself and others. It is a journey of deep personal growth and understanding, a pathway to a fulfilling life enriched with compassion and nurtured through self-care.

Chapter 4: Zen Meditation and Stress Reduction.

The Science Behind Zen Meditation or

The proof is in the pudding

As we transition to examining the application of evolved awareness, through Zen meditation in healthcare, we amplify focus on the recent studies and trends in healthcare that have started to embrace mindfulness as a therapeutic tool. It is here we outline how mindfulness, a pivotal aspect of Zen meditation, can be effectively utilized in healthcare settings to augment the mental well-being of patients, potentially aiding in faster recovery and better management of chronic diseases. The section will present a meticulous breakdown of various hiding, focusing techniques derived from Zen meditation that are being incorporated into healthcare, emphasizing their efficacy and benefits as depicted in scientific studies.

Meditation Techniques for Emotional Balance

Drawing focus on meditation techniques dedicated to achieving emotional balance, this segment envisions the current applications and potential future trajectories of these techniques in healthcare. The scientific literature has a growing body of evidence supporting the role of Zen meditation in fostering emotional balance, enhancing patient care, and reducing healthcare provider burnout. This part aims to offer a detailed insight into the scientific validations that underscore the adoption of these techniques in healthcare settings, presenting a comprehensive view of their benefits backed by empirical data.

Next, we discuss the facilitation of empathic communication through Zen practices within healthcare settings. This section leans heavily on recent studies to narrate how Zen meditation can nurture empathic communication between healthcare providers and patients, potentially fostering a more understanding and compassionate healthcare environment. It will expound upon the cognitive and neurological pathways enhanced through Zen meditation, aiming to provide a grounded perspective on its role in bolstering empathic communication in healthcare.

As we conclude, we focus on community building through Zen meditation and its prospective role in healthcare. We aim to detail the initiatives and programs that are paving the way for a more communal approach in healthcare, building support systems through Zen meditation groups and fostering environments that encourage mutual understanding and compassionate care. We draw upon case studies and pilot programs that have successfully integrated community-driven Zen meditation initiatives in healthcare settings.

The integration of Zen meditation in healthcare stands as a promising frontier with immense potential to revolutionize care delivery and patient outcomes. Through a detailed exploration grounded in the latest scientific research and trends, this comprehensive narrative delineates the current roles and the expansive prospects of incorporating Zen meditation into healthcare. It positions Zen meditation as a potent tool, backed by an ever-growing body of scientific validation, ready to forge a healthcare future steeped in compassion, understanding, and holistic well-being, presenting a healthcare landscape transformed through the nurturing principles of Zen meditation. This exploration stands as an invitation to healthcare stakeholders to delve deeper into the enriching potentials that Zen meditation holds for a more compassionate, empathetic, and effective healthcare system.

Progressing further, we will explore the realms of mindfulness through guided meditation scripts. These scripts are crafted meticulously to introduce healthcare professionals to the art of staying present and fully engaging with the here and now. Through carefully crafted narratives, we will guide individuals to focus on their breath, sensations, and the surrounding environment, encouraging a mindfulness practice that can be a cornerstone in reducing stress and fostering well-being in the hectic healthcare setting.

In this segment, we will furnish healthcare professionals with scripts aimed at fostering emotional balance. Through a series of guided narratives, professionals will be guided to find their center, maintain balance in the face of challenges, and cultivate a serene mind. These scripts will entail grounding exercises, visualizations, and affirmations to facilitate a state of emotional harmony, equipping healthcare professionals with the tools to navigate the demanding landscapes of their profession with grace and balance.

Advancing the theme of empathic communication, this section will offer scripts to aid healthcare professionals in nurturing empathy and understanding in their interactions. Through these scripts, individuals will be guided to envisage scenarios where empathy takes the front seat, enhancing their ability to relate to patients and peers empathically, and fostering a work environment grounded in understanding and mutual respect.

Self-Compassion Narratives: Guided Scripts for Self-Care

Transitioning into the nurturing embrace of self-compassion, we will present a series of guided meditation scripts centered on self-care and kindness towards oneself. These narratives will guide healthcare professionals in developing a kind, understanding relationship with themselves, encouraging moments of pause, reflection, and self-nurturance, thereby fostering a reservoir of self-compassion to draw from in challenging times.

Concluding our exploration, we will present scripts aimed at building a sense of community and unity among healthcare teams. Through guided group meditations and team-building narratives, these scripts will foster a spirit of collaboration and mutual support, encouraging healthcare professionals to work harmoniously, respecting and uplifting each other in the pursuit of providing excellent healthcare.

This comprehensive guide to developing guided meditation scripts stands as a beacon of support for healthcare professionals. Through a rich exploration of various themes ranging from mindfulness to community building, these scripts aim to offer a nurturing space, encouraging professionals to cultivate inner harmony, empathy, and resilience. Each script is designed with the utmost care, drawing from the rich traditions of meditation and mindfulness, aiming to offer solace, a space of tranquility amidst the bustling environment of healthcare settings, guiding professionals to foster a healthcare environment grounded in compassion, understanding, and holistic well-being. This guide invites healthcare professionals to immerse themselves in these nurturing narratives, embarking on a journey towards a more compassionate, balanced, and harmonious self.

Here are some examples of Scripts

Script 1:

Find a quiet and comfortable place to sit or lie down. Close your eyes and take deep, slow breaths, focusing on the sensation of the breath entering and leaving your body.

Visualize a tranquil scene — a forest, a beach, or a meadow. Place yourself in this scene and feel a sense of peace and calm enveloping you.

As you immerse yourself in this serene landscape, let go of any tensions, fears, or anxieties. Allow yourself to be filled with a sense of tranquility and well-being, being present in this moment of peace.

Script 2:

Sit comfortably in a quiet space. Close your eyes and focus on your breath, feeling the rhythm of your natural breathing pattern.

Imagine a gentle stream flowing in front of you. Visualize yourself placing any worries, fears, or tensions into leaves and letting them float away on the stream.

With each breath, allow more leaves to take away any burdens, leaving you feeling lighter and more peaceful with each moment.

Script 3:

Find a comfortable seat in a quiet space. Close your eyes and bring your attention to your breath, inhaling deeply and exhaling slowly.

Imagine a warm, golden light above you, filled with love and kindness. Visualize this light descending and enveloping you, filling you with warmth, love, and compassion.

Allow this golden light to heal any pains, soothe any worries, and fill you with a deep sense of peace and love for yourself and others.

Script 4:

Sit or lie down comfortably in a quiet space. Close your eyes and take deep breaths, feeling the air fill your lungs and then slowly leave your body.

Visualize a safe and sacred space around you, a place of unconditional love and acceptance. Imagine yourself in this space, filled with a sense of security and well-being.

As you dwell in this sacred space, allow yourself to release any tensions, fears, or anxieties, embracing a state of peace, love, and harmony.

Feel free to use these scripts in your meditation sessions. They are designed to help cultivate a peaceful and compassionate state of mind. Let me know if there is anything else you would like to explore.

Script 5:

Find a comfortable position in a quiet space. Close your eyes and take deep, nurturing breaths.

Picture a gentle, compassionate figure standing before you, enveloping you in a warm embrace. This figure embodies self-compassion, reminding you to treat yourself with the kindness and understanding you readily offer to others.

Inhale self-kindness and exhale self-criticism. Allow this figure to guide you in embracing yourself with compassion and understanding.

Script 6:

Sit or lay down comfortably. Focus your attention inward and take deep, nourishing breaths.

Visualize a garden within your heart, a place where self-love blooms with vibrant colors. With each breath, nurture this garden with kind thoughts, affirming your worth and acknowledging your efforts.

Allow yourself to dwell in this garden for a while, nourishing your inner self with love, kindness, and understanding.

Script 7:

Gather in a comfortable space with your team. Sit in a circle, and as you close your eyes, visualize a thread of light connecting each heart in the circle, forming a bond of unity and harmony.

Breathing in unity, breathing out harmony. Let yourselves feel the collective strength, the mutual support, and the shared goal of compassionate service.

Feel this connection deepening, fostering a community of respect, understanding, and cooperation.

Script 8:

In a quiet space with your team, sit comfortably, closing your eyes and focusing on your breath.

Imagine a circle of trust and cooperation surrounding you all, a safe space where each individual is seen, heard, and respected. Visualize this circle as a source of strength, a place where each member can draw support and inspiration.

Allow yourselves to dwell in this circle for a few moments, feeling the bonds of unity, trust, and mutual respect strengthening with each breath.

Script 9:

Find a quiet place to sit or lie down. Close your eyes and focus on your breath.

Visualize a protective shield around you, a shield made of compassion and understanding. Even amid chaos and pressure, this shield remains unbroken, maintaining a space of calm and compassion within you.

Breathe in calmness, and breathe out tension. Allow yourself to remain compassionate, centered, and calm, even under pressure.

Script 10:

In a peaceful setting, find a comfortable posture. Close your eyes and focus on your breath.

Imagine holding a compass in your hand, a compass that always points towards compassion. No matter the pressure and the stress, let this compass guide you to respond with understanding, kindness, and empathy.

Let yourself dwell in this space for a while, grounding yourself in the guiding principle of compassion, a principle that remains steadfast even under pressure.

Research consistently shows that meditation fosters mental resilience, helping individuals stay grounded amidst the chaos. A routine meditation practice can facilitate a clearer mind, enhancing focus and productivity by allowing individuals to work with a more centered and calm disposition.

Moreover, the consistent practice of meditation can cultivate mindfulness, a quality that encourages a heightened awareness of the present moment. This can translate into better decision-making in the workplace as it nurtures a space of clarity and focus, away from the noise and distractions that often accompany a hectic work environment.

A meditation routine can also serve as a powerful antidote to the stress and anxiety that is prevalent in high-pressure work settings. By promoting relaxation and helping to reduce cortisol levels, meditation can foster a greater sense of well-being and happiness, which not only benefits individuals but creates a more harmonious work environment.

Furthermore, adopting a meditation routine can enhance creativity and problem-solving skills. By encouraging a state of relaxation, meditation allows the mind to break free from rigid patterns of thinking, paving the way for innovative solutions and fresh perspectives to emerge.

Despite the apparent benefits, establishing a meditation routine in a hectic work environment requires dedication and perhaps a shift in organizational culture to prioritize employee well-being. This might include creating quiet spaces for meditation, encouraging breaks for mindfulness practices, and possibly incorporating guided meditation sessions to facilitate this health-promoting practice among employees.

As we focus on the development of a meditation routine, it is essential to approach it with flexibility and understanding. Some days might allow for a longer meditation session, while on busier days, even a few minutes of focused breathing can make a significant difference. The key is consistency, and over time, even a small daily practice can yield substantial benefits, creating a ripple effect of increased well-being and productivity in the workplace.

Creating a meditation routine in a hectic work environment stands as a cornerstone in nurturing a healthy, vibrant, and productive work life. It goes beyond just personal well-being, enhancing collaborative spirits, fostering creativity, and essentially, sculpting a workplace that thrives on understanding, empathy, and focused energy. It is not just an investment in personal health but a foundational element in building resilient, harmonious, and successful work environments.

Steps in cultivating meditation and practices or easy does it.

Start with short sessions. Begin with short meditation sessions, perhaps 5 to 10 minutes each day, and gradually increase the duration as you become more comfortable with the practice. This ensures that you do not feel overwhelmed and can easily fit meditation into your busy schedule.

Leverage technology. Utilize meditation apps and platforms that offer guided meditation sessions, which can be a great way to stay on track and maintain consistency in your meditation practice.

Create a serene space. Designate a quiet and comfortable space in your office or home where you can meditate without disturbances. This could be a small corner with a comfortable chair and calming accessories such as a plant or a soft cushion.

Integrate meditation into your routine. Try to integrate meditation into your existing routine, such as meditating during your commute (if you are not driving), during lunch breaks, or before meetings to ground yourself and clear your mind.

Breathing exercises. Learn simple breathing exercises that you can do anytime, anywhere. Focusing on your breath can be a quick way to center yourself and reduce stress.

Mindful moments. Practice mindfulness by taking short breaks throughout the day to focus fully on the present moment. This could involve focusing on your breath, the sensations in your body, or the sounds around you.

Walking meditations. If you find it challenging to sit still for a meditation session, try walking meditations. This involves walking slowly and mindfully, paying attention to each step and your surroundings and can be a great way to incorporate meditation into a busy day.

Gratitude practice. Start or end your day with a gratitude practice, where you take a few moments to reflect on the things that you are thankful for. This can shift your mindset and promote a positive outlook.

Visualization. Engage in visualization techniques where you imagine a peaceful and calm place or visualize completing a task. This can be a powerful tool to reduce anxiety and enhance focus.

Seek support. If possible, create a meditation group with your colleagues or friends to encourage each other and stay accountable in your meditation practice.

Be patient with yourself. Understand that meditation is a skill that takes time to develop. Be patient with yourself and approach your practice with a sense of curiosity and openness.

The Creation of Meditation Spaces in Healthcare Centers. Some examples.

Patients and their families find a haven in these spots, where they can pause, breathe, and sometimes find a much-needed emotional release. For example, the All Children's Hospital in St. Petersburg, Florida has a sanctuary space where families can find a moment of peace amid the hospital hustle and bustle.

Healthcare providers can recharge in these areas, taking a few minutes between their hectic schedules to ground themselves, ensuring they approach their work with fresh eyes and a calm mind.

Design

Natural Elements: Many hospitals are moving towards greener designs. The Khoo Teck Puat Hospital in Singapore is a notable example, offering natural ventilation, lush gardens, and even a waterfall, fostering a tranquil atmosphere.

Color Scheme: Some hospitals adopt a vibrant color scheme to lighten the mood and foster positivity. The Children's Hospital in Pittsburgh offers individual rooms painted in vibrant colors, fostering a friendly environment, especially for young patients.

Furniture: Furniture that offers comfort and homeliness is key. The Maggie's Centres across the UK have been designed with a homely and welcoming aesthetic, creating a comforting space for cancer patients and their families.

Art: Incorporating art is a growing trend in healthcare. The Cleveland Clinic has its contemporary art collection to foster a healing environment, including visual arts, music, dance, and more.

Lighting: Utilizing a well-thought-out lighting scheme can have a calming effect. The Elisabeth Severance Prentiss Center in Cleveland has been designed with large windows allowing natural light to flood the space, creating a warm atmosphere.

Quiet: Establishing a quiet space is vital for meditation. The Ronald Reagan UCLA Medical Center in Los Angeles houses a 'healing garden,' providing a silent retreat amidst natural surroundings.

Accessibility: Ensuring accessibility for all individuals is key. The UCSF Medical Center at Mission Bay in San Francisco features meditation rooms and rooftop gardens that are accessible to everyone, including individuals with disabilities.

I very much encourage the reader to do an Internet search for these particular clinics that were listed above. Due to copyright requirements, etc. I was not able to post the photos. They are amazing. These clinics are utopian, wonderful architectural, displays of excellence and provide optimal environments for healing.

Here are some suggested architectural scenarios

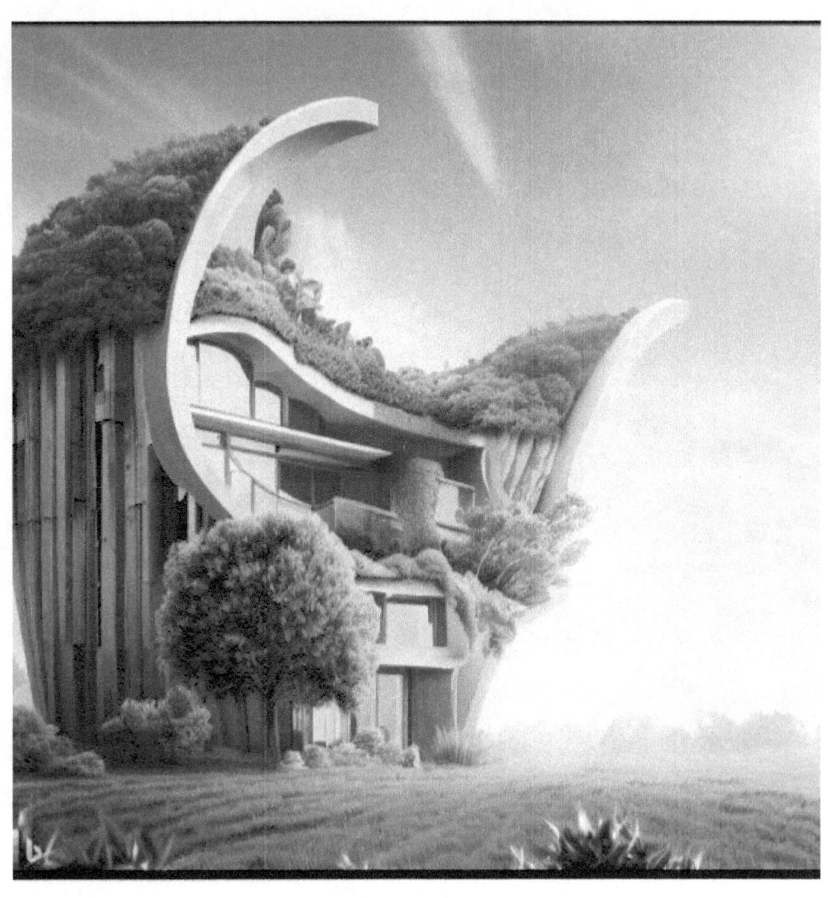

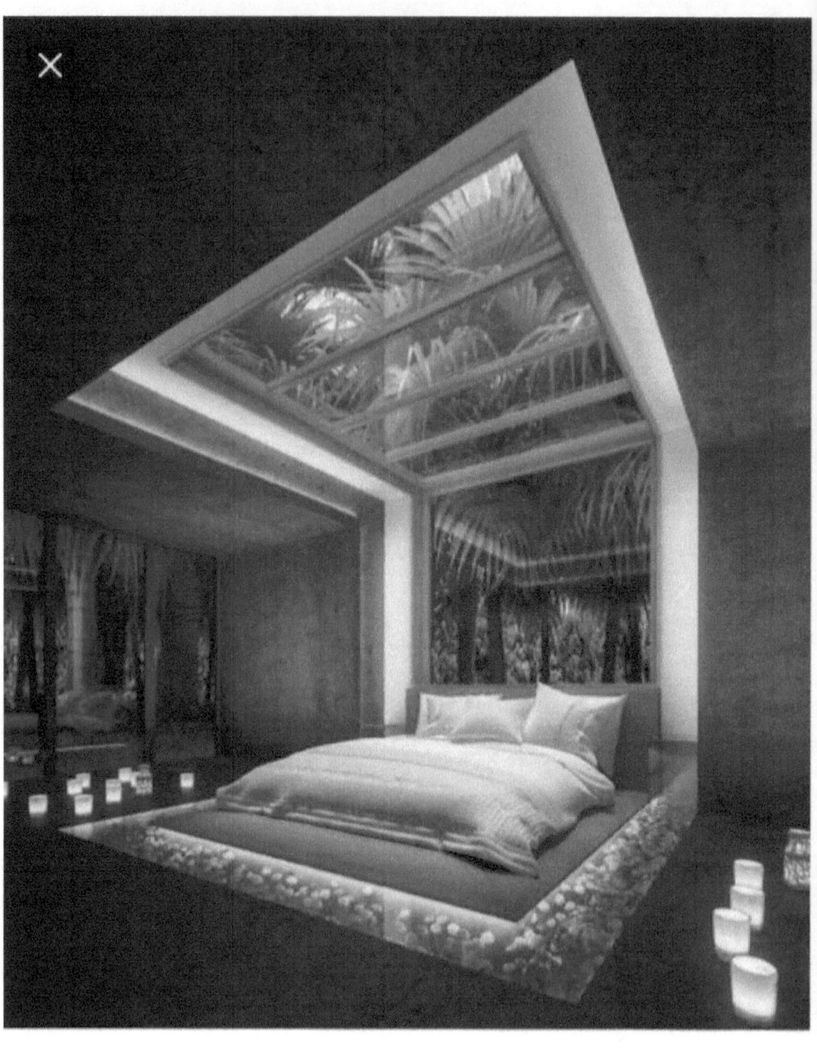

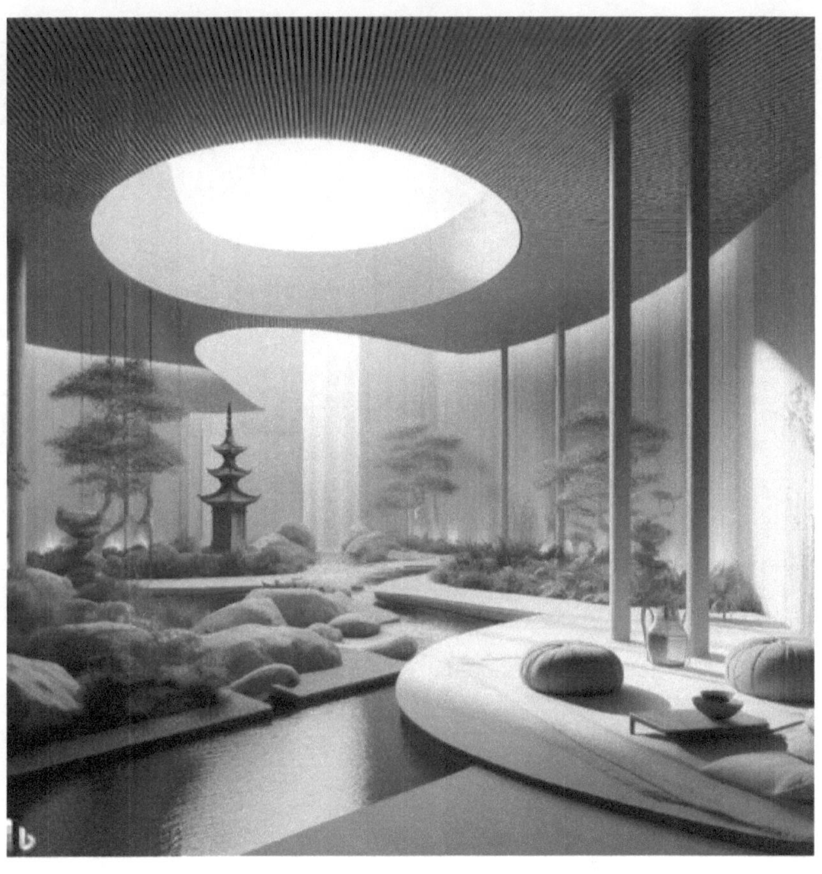

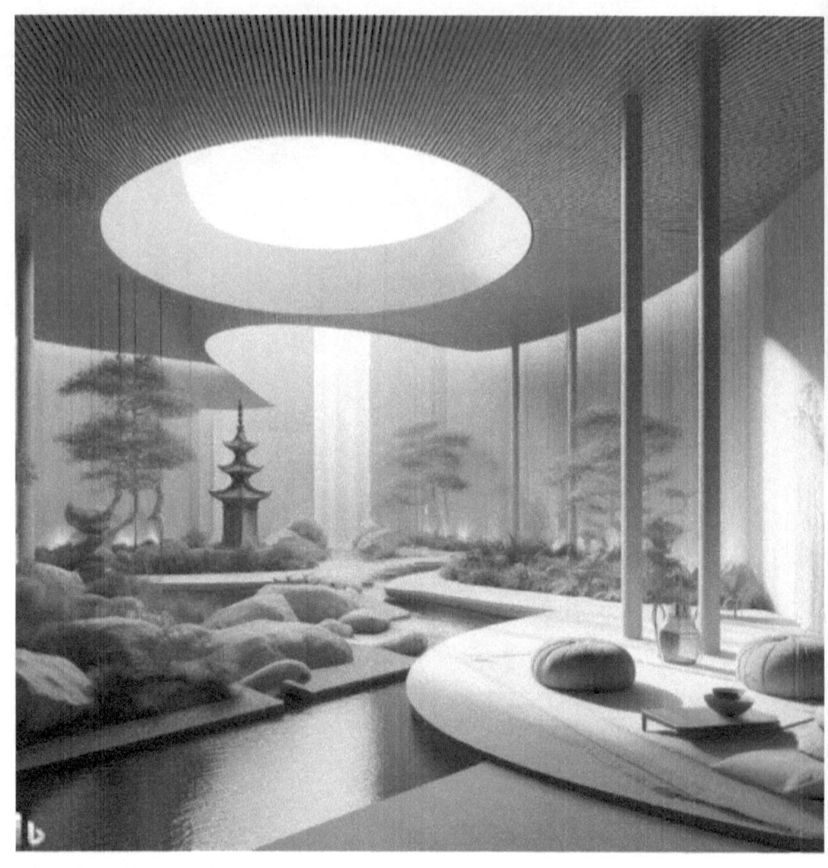

Conducting Meditation

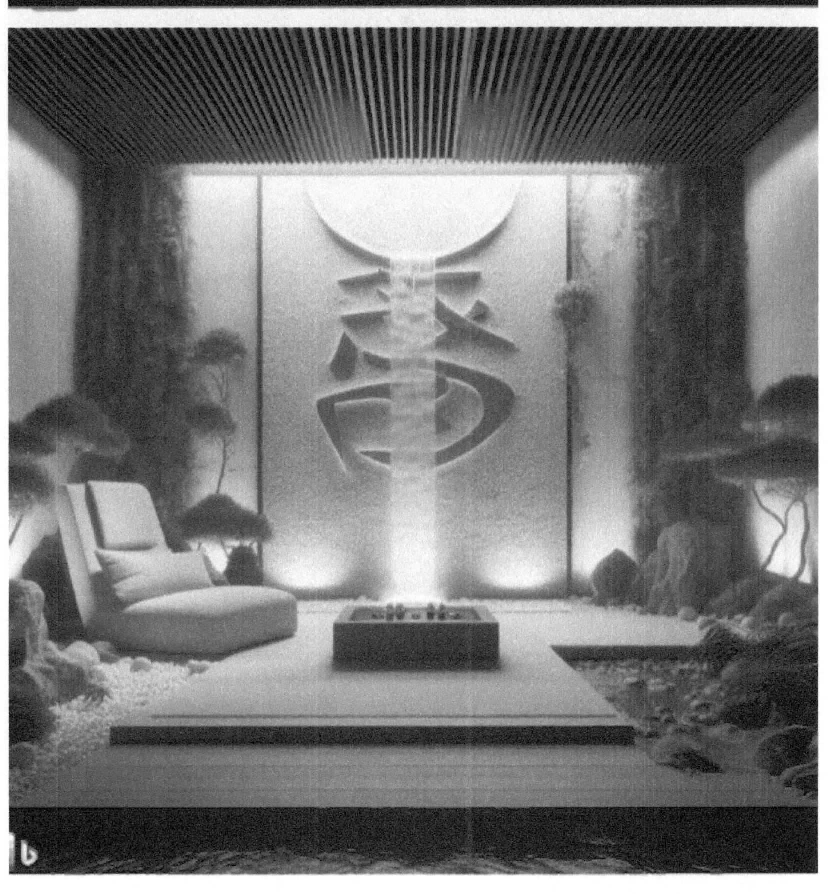

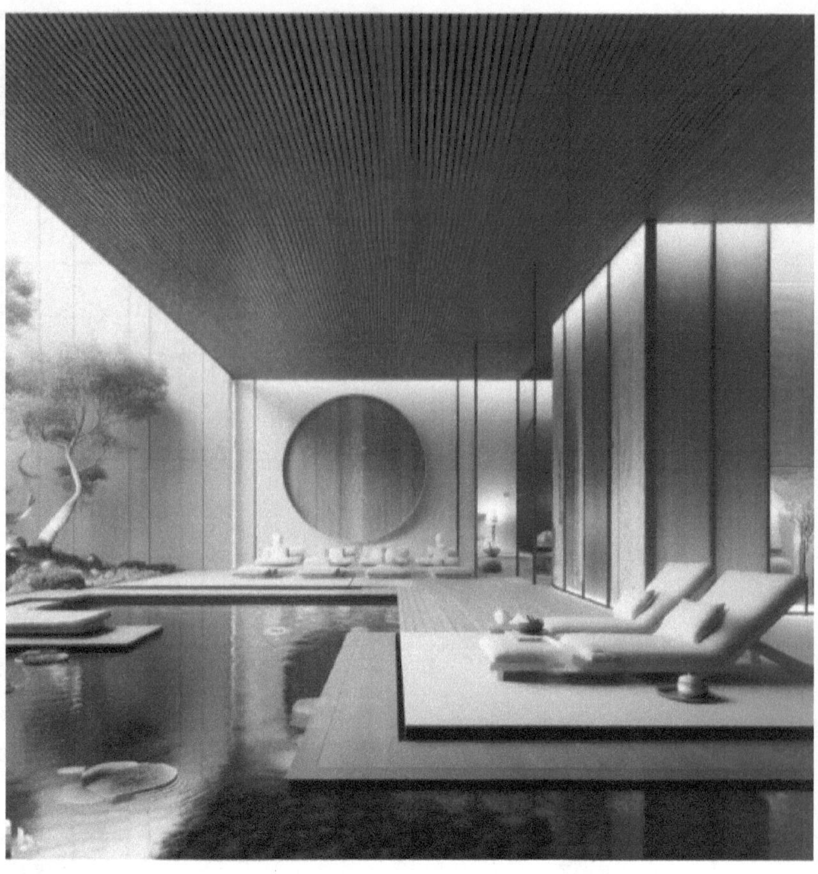

Creating a guided space for meditation is equally important in aiding the healing process.

Guided Meditation: Institutions like the University

of Michigan Rogel Cancer Center offers guided meditation sessions to help patients, families, and staff manage stress more effectively.

Self-Guided Meditation: Providing resources for self-guided meditation is vital. Stanford Health Care has meditation podcasts available on its website, allowing individuals to meditate at their convenience.

Resource Material: Offering material that assists in meditation, such as books or apps, can be beneficial. The Mayo Clinic offers a range of resources including books and videos to facilitate meditation.

Regular Schedule: Many healthcare centers have designated schedules for meditation. Massachusetts General Hospital has a Benson-Henry Institute which hosts regular meditation sessions, promoting a routine for individuals to follow.

Feedback and Adjustments: Taking feedback from users and making necessary adjustments to improve the environment continually is vital. Many institutions seek feedback through regular surveys to understand the users' needs better.

The Importance of a Healing Environment: Psychological Perspectives
    Understanding the Concept

A healing environment goes beyond the physical attributes of a healthcare setting. It encompasses a space that supports the psychological well-being of individuals, promoting a sense of safety, tranquility, and peace.

By creating a calming and nurturing space, healthcare settings can significantly reduce the stress and anxiety levels of patients, families, and staff members. Hospitals that foster a healing environment pay attention to every detail, including the choice of colors, materials, and lighting, which can all evoke a sense of calm and positivity.

Improved Mental Health

The psychological state of an individual can drastically improve in a healing environment. Spaces designed with the wellness of the individual in mind foster better mental health by reducing factors that can lead to depression or anxiety.

Healing environments facilitate faster recovery. From a psychological standpoint, when patients are comfortable and at ease, it aids in quicker recovery as they can rest more efficiently, aiding in the recuperation process.

Therapeutic Gardens

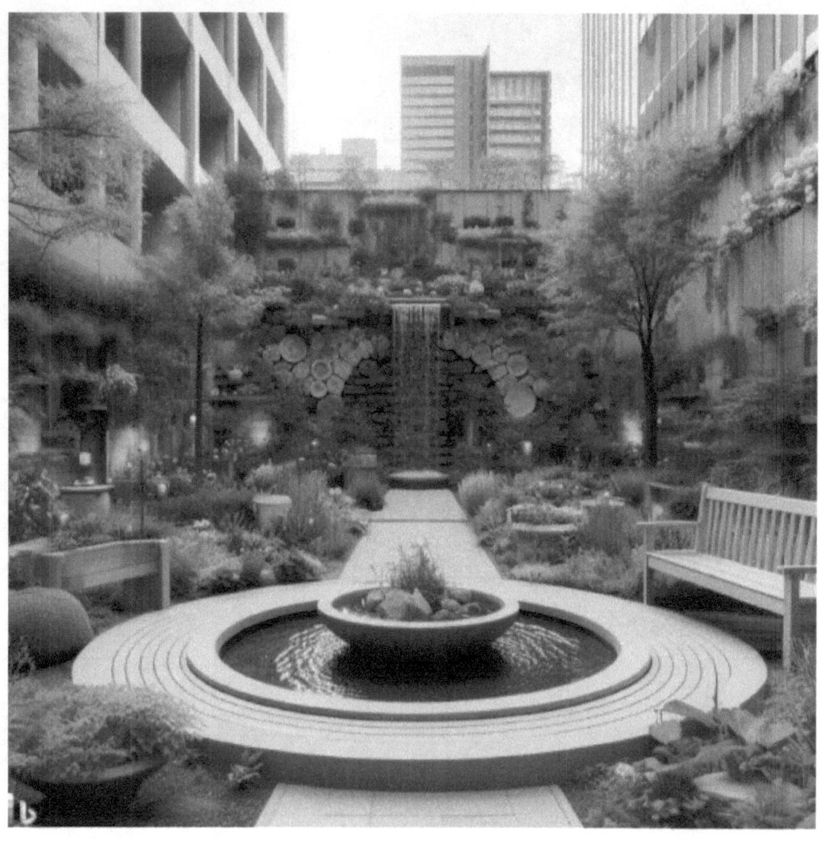

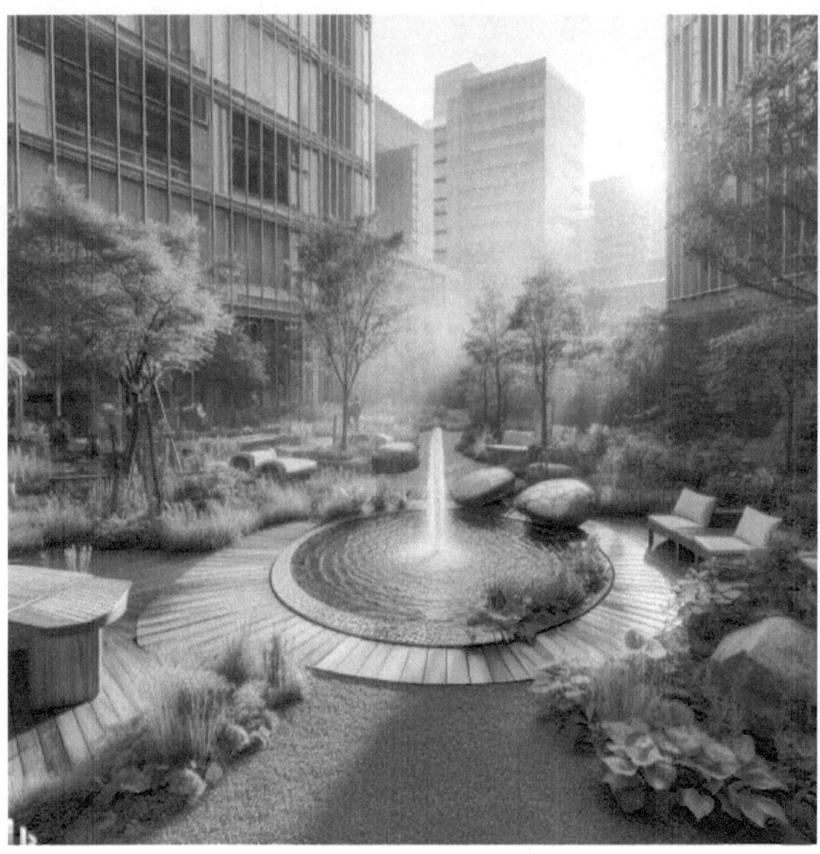

Therapeutic gardens can have a profound impact on a patient's psychological health. The healing power of being in touch with nature can not be underestimated. Hospitals are increasingly incorporating therapeutic gardens to enhance the healing process.

Natural light has been shown to have numerous psychological benefits. It can improve mood, create a sense of openness, and reduce feelings of confinement, which is particularly beneficial in healthcare settings.

Art therapy is gaining traction as a tool in healing environments. Art installations or spaces for artistic creation can provide a therapeutic outlet for patients, aiding in emotional expression and mental healing.

Having aesthetically pleasing environments can foster a positive outlook. Consideration of the art, color schemes, and overall aesthetics of a place can play a significant role in healing from a psychological perspective.

Creating soundscapes that are soothing rather than irritating can have a significant impact on the psychological well-being of individuals in healthcare settings. Sounds that mimic nature, for instance, can have a calming effect.

Utilizing aromatherapy in healthcare settings can potentially create a more calming and pleasant atmosphere, addressing the psychological aspects of healing through the sense of smell.

Conclusion

Understanding and implementing the facets of a healing environment from a psychological perspective can significantly enhance the well-being of individuals in healthcare settings. It's a multi-dimensional approach that goes beyond physical healing, offering a holistic pathway to recovery that encompasses mind, body, and spirit.

This overview should give a comprehensive understanding of the psychological perspectives revolving around healing environments. Let me know if you'd like to delve deeper into any of these aspects.

How the Environment Influences Healing: A Psychological Perspective

Introduction

Healing involves more than just physical recovery; it is profoundly influenced by the psychological well-being of individuals. The environment in which this healing takes place can either foster or hinder psychological recovery. Here, we delve into various elements of the environment and how they can influence healing from a psychological standpoint.

Creating environments that promote psychological safety can foster trust and openness, encouraging individuals to express themselves without fear of reprisal, thereby aiding in the healing process.

Environments that offer comfort and facilitate ease can go a long way in reducing stress and promoting a positive psychological state, crucial for healing. Elements such as ergonomic furniture and tranquil spaces play pivotal roles here.

Incorporation of Natural Elements

Biophilic design, which involves bringing elements of the natural world into built environments, can enhance healing. It recognizes the inherent human affinity for nature and utilizes it to create spaces that are psychologically comforting and healing.

Providing green spaces in healthcare settings can create a haven of peace and tranquility, offering respite and encouraging a more positive psychological state, essential for the healing journey.

The Role of Art

Art can serve as a comforting and uplifting presence in healthcare environments. Paintings, sculptures, and other art installations can provide visual stimuli that ignite positive emotions and facilitate psychological healing.

Instituting therapeutic art programs can offer patients an outlet for expression, helping them work through psychological barriers and find a pathway to healing through creativity.

Harmonized Sound Environment

Creating an environment with a harmonized sound profile, where irritating noises are minimized, can offer a psychologically comforting space that promotes healing.

Spaces for Reflection

Meditation Spaces

Establishing dedicated spaces for meditation can foster deep reflection and inner peace, which are vital for psychological healing.

Quiet Rooms

Creating quiet rooms where individuals can escape the noise and chaos to find moments of peace can foster psychological healing, providing a sanctuary for reflection and calm.

Conclusion

From a psychological standpoint, the environment holds a substantial influence over the healing process. Understanding and integrating psychological principles into the design and operation of healthcare environments can create spaces that not only heal the body but also nurture the mind, promoting holistic healing and well-being.

Feel free to reach out if there are any other aspects you'd like to explore or discuss.

How the Healing Environment Influences Recovery Rates: A Statistical Overview

Introduction

The influence of healing environments on the recovery rates of patients has become a focal point in recent research. In this overview, we will delve deep into various studies and present statistical data showcasing how different elements of a healing environment have impacted recovery rates over the years.

Literature Review some samples of the use of therapeutic instruments in real-time and architecture

The Impact of Natural Elements

An area that has witnessed considerable attention is the role of natural elements in the healing process.

Biophilic Design: One significant study in this domain was conducted by Ulrich in 1984, which documented that patients having a view of natural scenery from their rooms had a faster recovery rate, experiencing an 8.5% reduction in hospital stay compared to those without such views.

Green Spaces: A further study published in the "Environmental Science & Technology Journal" in 2010 highlighted that individuals with higher exposure to green spaces had a 28% lower risk of developing mental health issues, showcasing the therapeutic benefits of being close to nature.

Art has emerged as a pivotal therapeutic tool in healthcare settings.

Therapeutic Art Programs: Stuckey & Nobel 2010 highlighted the role of art programs in healing environments, noting a substantial 28% reduction in requests for pain medication in hospitals that integrated art programs into their healing approach.

Sensory Considerations

A considerable portion of research has focused on the sensory elements and their role in promoting healing.

Aromatherapy: The introduction of aromatherapy in the healthcare setting was analyzed in a study in 2014 by Fayazi et al., which documented a significant drop in patient anxiety scores, witnessing a reduction rate of up to 50%.

Sound Environment: The sound environment in healthcare settings has also come under scrutiny. A study by Huisman et al., in 2012 reported that hospitals that maintained a harmonized sound environment saw an improvement of 47% in patient sleep patterns, which is a crucial factor in the healing process.

Spaces for Reflection

Spaces designated for reflection have demonstrated considerable benefits in enhancing recovery rates.

Meditation Spaces: A study published in the "Archives of Internal Medicine" in 2012 emphasized the role of meditation in reducing heart disease risk by 48%, underscoring the necessity of having spaces dedicated to meditation in healthcare settings.

Quiet Rooms: Marcus and Barnes in 1999 highlighted the positive impact of quiet rooms in healthcare settings, associating them with a 40% reduction in stress levels among patients and healthcare workers, thus facilitating better recovery outcomes.

Conclusion

The detailed statistical data from various studies unequivocally underscore the monumental role that a well-designed healing environment plays in improving recovery rates. The compelling figures present a strong case for the integral role of nurturing environments in fostering not only a quicker recovery but also a more effective one. Therefore, it is imperative for healthcare facilities to prioritize the creation of healing environments, backed by empirical data, to enhance the well-being and recovery rates of patients.

Introduction to Zen architectural design and a call for architects to incorporate the style into their planning especially that of healthcare environments. Let us begin.

In the realm of architectural design, the influence of Zen principles is markedly noticeable, grounding designs in concepts of simplicity, natural elements, and the proficient utilization of space. Architects adhering to these principles endeavor to form spaces that resonate with peace, tranquility, and harmony. This discourse seeks to elucidate the paramount roles played by space and simplicity, fundamental tenets in Zen-inspired architectural design.

Zen Principles in Architectural Design: An Exploration

Simplicity, commonly referred to as Kanso in the Zen philosophy, advocates for the omission of the non-essential, thereby highlighting the inherent beauty of materials and structures.

Ah, understood. "Kanso" (◇◇) is a Japanese term and concept derived from Zen thought, particularly in the realm of aesthetics and design. It translates roughly to "simplicity" or "elimination of clutter." Kanso emphasizes the idea that beauty and utility need not be overstated or ornate, but rather can be found in the simple, clear, and concise.

In architecture and interior design, Kanso can be observed in:

Minimalist Designs

Structures and spaces that eliminate unnecessary elements and emphasize the essential function of a building. This means clean lines, unadorned walls, and a focus on functional elements.

Open Spaces

A clear sense of flow and openness in a room or building, avoiding clutter and excessive decoration. This is commonly seen in traditional Japanese homes where rooms can have multiple functions and are transformed by moving simple screens or panels.

Use of Natural Materials

Using materials in their natural or lightly finished state. Think of wood that still shows its grain or stone that bears the marks of its quarrying.

Subtle Beauty

Details or elements that might not scream for attention but provide a deep sense of beauty or utility upon closer inspection.

Examples worldwide incorporating Kanso

Traditional Japanese Homes

As mentioned earlier, traditional Japanese homes often embody the principle of Kanso with their open spaces, tatami mats, and multipurpose rooms divided by sliding screens.

The "Tiny House" Movement

Found predominantly in Western countries, these homes emphasize living simply and with only what one needs. The interiors are often functional and devoid of excess.

Scandinavian Design

Though not Japanese, the Nordic design principle aligns closely with Kanso. It emphasizes clean lines, functionality, and minimalism, evident in brands like IKEA or Danish furniture design.

Modern Architectural Movements

Many contemporary buildings, especially those under the modern or minimalistic architectural style, reflect Kanso by emphasizing simple geometric shapes, open spaces, and a lack of ornate detailing.

Zen Gardens

While not a "building," these gardens are a testament to the Kanso aesthetic, utilizing rocks, gravel, and sparse plantings to create serene landscapes.

In essence, Kanso reminds us of the elegance of simplicity and the power of the understated. It's an approach to design and living that can lead to a clearer, more focused experience of space and structure.

The choice of materials is pivotal in the evocation of a serene atmosphere. Simplicity is championed through the use of natural, unpretentious, and understated materials which foster a tranquil environment.

Color Selection

A careful selection of the color palette is equally vital. Soft, neutral shades including whites and beiges are preferred, steering clear of loud, vibrant colors. This choice engenders a soothing effect, allowing the inherent beauty of the environment to shine through, unmasked by distracting hues.

Spatial Configuration in Zen Design

The Zen philosophy extends its influence to spatial configurations, where space isn't just a physical entity but holds metaphorical significance too.

Open Layouts

Open layouts are a distinctive feature, promoting a seamless flow and free movement within the space. The uninterrupted spatial arrangement encourages interaction and connectivity, fostering a harmonious ambiance.

Functional Use of Space

Functionality is at the heart of Zen-inspired spaces. Every element incorporated has a designated purpose, sidestepping unnecessary clutter and encouraging a simplistic approach that is both efficient and aesthetically pleasing.

Real-World Implementations of Zen Principles

Numerous real-world examples echo the successful implementation of Zen principles in architectural designs.

The Katsura Imperial Villa

The Katsura Imperial Villa in Japan stands as a testament to the seamless integration of Zen principles in architectural endeavors, beautifully marrying simplicity and spatial intelligence to offer a tranquil retreat.

Tadao Ando's Contributions

In a more contemporary setting, architect Tadao Ando's body of work showcases a profound influence of Zen principles. He harmonizes natural elements and simplicity, weaving them into designs that offer tranquility and are innately peaceful.

Conclusion

The Zen principles of space and simplicity have been guiding lights in the field of architectural design, ushering in designs that are not just visually pleasing but also echo with tranquility and foster well-being. They teach us the art of marrying functionality with aesthetics, where every element serves a purpose, and the natural beauty of materials is allowed to shine through. The focus is on creating harmonious spaces, that serve as a sanctuary of calm and peace in a fast-paced world, offering individuals a space to reconnect with themselves and with nature.

By immersing ourselves in the Zen philosophy, we learn the invaluable lesson of harmony, both with ourselves and with the environments we inhabit. It encourages architects to think beyond the physicality of spaces and to embrace the spiritual, offering designs that are not just structures but experiences that echo with tranquility and peace.

Zen Principles in Architectural Design: Cultivating Harmony Through Simplicity and Natural Materials

Introduction

In the realm of architectural design, the profound influence of Zen principles is strikingly evident, anchoring designs in the fundamental concepts of simplicity, natural elements, and the proficient utilization of space. Architects who embrace these principles endeavor to craft spaces that resonate with peace, tranquility, and harmony. This discourse seeks to illuminate the paramount roles played by space and simplicity, the core tenets of Zen-inspired architectural design.

Zen Philosophy: A Foundation of Harmony

Zen philosophy, rooted in Japanese Buddhism, forms the philosophical bedrock of Zen-inspired architectural design. At its core, Zen advocates for mindfulness, simplicity, and the pursuit of inner peace. These principles profoundly shape architectural endeavors, resulting in spaces that evoke a sense of calm and balance.

Material Choices

The selection of materials is pivotal in creating a serene atmosphere. Zen-inspired architects favor natural, unpretentious, and understated materials such as wood, stone, and paper. These materials, in their purest forms, evoke a sense of harmony with nature.

Color Selection

A careful choice of the color palette is equally vital. Zen spaces predominantly feature soft, neutral shades including whites, beiges, and muted earth tones. The absence of loud, vibrant colors fosters a soothing effect, allowing the inherent beauty of the environment to shine through, unmasked by distracting hues.

Natural Elements: A Source of Tranquility

In Zen-inspired architectural design, a profound connection with nature is pivotal. The incorporation of natural elements serves to enhance the sense of harmony and tranquility within spaces.

Integration of Nature

Zen gardens, indoor courtyards, and large windows that frame natural vistas are common elements. These features bring the outdoors inside, creating a seamless connection with the natural world.

Use of Water

The inclusion of water features, such as ponds or fountains, is emblematic of Zen design. The gentle flow of water symbolizes serenity and life, further reinforcing the harmonious atmosphere.

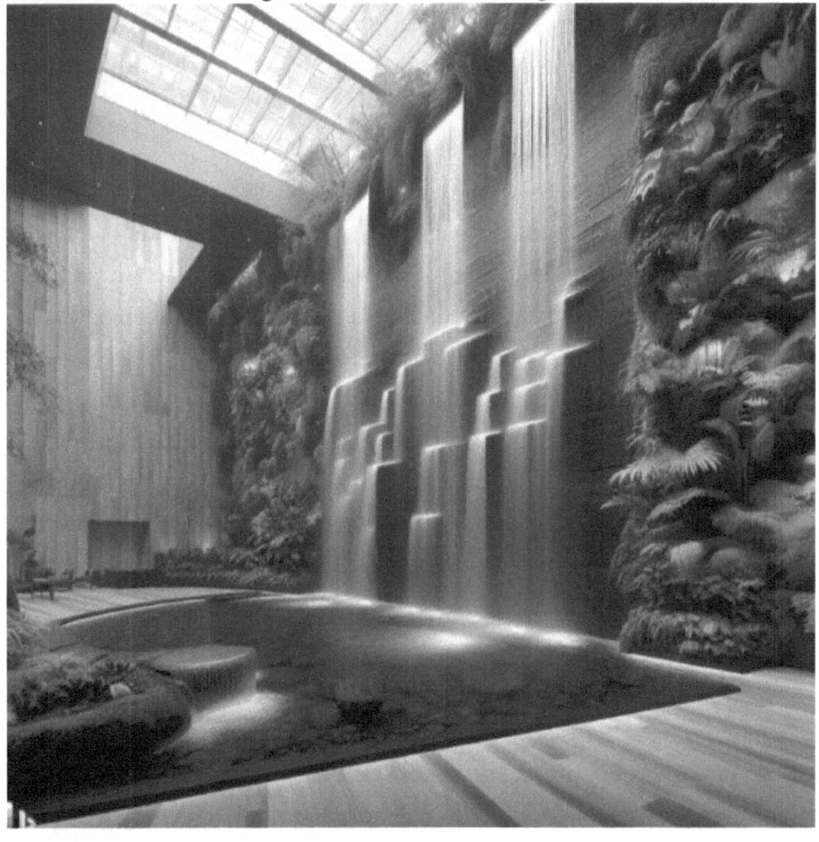

Spatial Configuration: Beyond the Physical

Zen philosophy extends its influence to spatial configurations, where space isn't just a physical entity but holds metaphorical significance.

Open Layouts

Open layouts are a distinctive feature, promoting a seamless flow and free movement within the space. The uninterrupted spatial arrangement encourages interaction and connectivity, fostering a harmonious ambiance.

Functional Use of Space

Functionality is at the heart of Zen-inspired spaces. Every element incorporated has a designated purpose, sidestepping unnecessary clutter and encouraging a simplistic approach that is both efficient and aesthetically pleasing.

Real-World Exemplars of Zen Principles

The Katsura Imperial Villa

Situated in Japan, the Katsura Imperial Villa stands as a testament to the seamless integration of Zen principles in architectural endeavors. It beautifully marries simplicity and spatial intelligence to offer a tranquil retreat immersed in natural beauty.

Tadao Ando's Contributions

In a more contemporary setting, architect Tadao Ando's body of work showcases a profound influence of Zen principles. He harmonizes natural elements and simplicity, weaving them into designs that offer tranquility and innate peace.

Additional Examples

The Ryoan-ji Temple Rock Garden (Kyoto, Japan): This iconic Zen garden exemplifies the power of simplicity, featuring a meticulously raked gravel garden with 15 carefully placed rocks. Its minimalist design invites contemplation and reflection.

Fallingwater (Mill Run, Pennsylvania, USA): Architect Frank Lloyd Wright's Fallingwater seamlessly integrates with its natural surroundings. Its cantilevered design over a waterfall embodies Zen principles of harmony with nature.

The Church of Light (Osaka, Japan): Designed by Tadao Ando, this minimalist church employs natural light as a key element, creating a serene space that encourages spiritual reflection.

Conclusion: Crafting Spaces of Harmony

The Zen principles of space and simplicity have been guiding lights in the field of architectural design, ushering in designs that are not just visually pleasing but also echo with tranquility and foster well-being. They teach us the art of marrying functionality with aesthetics, where every element serves a purpose, and the natural beauty of materials is allowed to shine through. The focus is on creating harmonious spaces, that serve as a sanctuary of calm and peace in a fast-paced world, offering individuals a space to reconnect with themselves and with nature.

By immersing ourselves in the Zen philosophy, we learn the invaluable lesson of harmony, both with ourselves and with the environments we inhabit. It encourages architects to think beyond the physicality of spaces and to embrace the spiritual, offering designs that are not just structures but experiences that echo with tranquility and peace. In this union of Zen principles and architectural design, we find a profound synergy that elevates spaces into realms of serene beauty and balance.

The Impact on Patient Well-Being

Extensive research supports the idea that incorporating natural elements into healthcare environments has a profound impact on patient well-being:

Faster Recovery: Patients in rooms with views of nature tend to recover more quickly from surgery and illness, requiring less pain medication and experiencing fewer post-operative complications.

Stress Reduction: Exposure to natural elements reduces stress and anxiety levels, leading to improved patient outcomes. Lower stress levels can also enhance the immune system's function.

Enhanced Mental Health: Nature-inspired spaces promote positive mental health by reducing feelings of depression and increasing overall patient satisfaction with their care.

The Benefits for Medical Staff

It's not just patients who benefit from the integration of natural elements in healthcare environments; medical staff also experience positive effects:

Reduced Burnout: Healthcare professionals working in environments with natural elements report lower levels of burnout and improved job satisfaction. These environments provide a sense of respite and rejuvenation for staff.

Better Focus and Creativity: Exposure to nature at work can enhance staff focus and creativity, ultimately improving the quality of patient care.

Conclusion: Nature's Healing Touch

Incorporating natural elements into healthcare environments harnesses the healing power of nature, benefiting both patients and medical staff. From increased patient satisfaction and faster recovery to reduced stress and burnout among healthcare professionals, the impact is extensive. As healthcare design continues to evolve, the integration of nature's elements is proving to be a transformative approach that aligns with the innate human connection to the natural world. It offers a glimpse into a future where healthcare environments are not only places of healing but also spaces of profound well-being, harmony, and connection with the healing power of nature.

Healing Gardens: Bringing Nature into Healthcare

Introduction

In the realm of healthcare design, the profound influence of healing gardens and the integration of nature into healthcare settings is increasingly evident. This transformative approach recognizes the therapeutic benefits of nature and its capacity to promote healing and well-being. Architects and healthcare professionals are actively embracing the idea of creating healing gardens and incorporating natural elements to enhance patient outcomes and improve the working environment for medical staff. This discourse seeks to delve deeper into the multifaceted impact of healing gardens and the integration of nature within healthcare facilities, shedding light on their positive effects on both patients and medical staff.

Benefits for Medical Staff

The advantages of healing gardens and nature integration extend beyond patients and positively impact medical staff:

Reduced Burnout: Healthcare professionals who have access to healing gardens experience lower levels of burnout and increased job satisfaction. These spaces provide moments of respite and rejuvenation amid the demanding and often emotionally taxing nature of their roles. The opportunity to step into a healing garden can serve as a form of self-care for healthcare providers, helping them better manage stress and maintain their well-being.

Enhanced Well-Being: Exposure to natural elements at work fosters staff well-being, leading to improved focus, creativity, and ultimately better patient care. Medical staff who can take short breaks in healing gardens are more likely to return to their duties with a refreshed mindset, contributing to a more positive and effective healthcare environment.

Conclusion: Nature's Therapeutic Presence

Incorporating healing gardens and the integration of nature into healthcare environments harnesses the therapeutic power of nature, benefiting both patients and medical staff. From reduced stress and faster recovery times for patients to improved well-being and job satisfaction for healthcare professionals, the impact is substantial. This approach aligns with the profound human connection to the natural world and offers a vision of healthcare environments that prioritize not only physical healing but also holistic well-being. It underscores the therapeutic presence of nature as a fundamental element in healthcare design, offering spaces that promote healing, relaxation, and a sense of calm amid the challenges of healthcare settings. As healthcare design continues to evolve, the importance of healing gardens and the integration of nature is becoming increasingly evident, providing a blueprint for the future of patient-centered and staff-supportive healthcare facilities.

Concrete examples of Zen incorporation

Singapore's Gardens by the Bay

In Singapore, the Gardens by the Bay project showcases an exemplary embodiment of a healing garden. With its Flower Dome, Cloud Forest, and Supertree Grove, it offers a space where visitors can immerse themselves in a rich botanical environment and experience healing through a close interaction with nature.

The Therapeutic Garden in HortPark, Singapore

Also in Singapore, the Therapeutic Garden in HortPark has been designed with therapeutic landscapes to offer emotional and psychological healing. The space is known for its calming effects, providing a therapeutic escape amid urban settings.

Portland's Legacy Emanuel Medical Center Healing Garden

Across the Pacific in Portland, Oregon, the Legacy Emanuel Medical Center has established a healing garden that offers patients, families, and staff a serene environment to find comfort and peace. The garden features paths for reflective walks, seating areas, and water features, creating a tranquil setting that encourages healing.

United Kingdom's Horatio's Garden

In the United Kingdom, Horatio's Garden creates beautiful and therapeutic gardens in NHS spinal injury centers. They have a handful of projects across the UK, each offering a sanctuary for spinal injury patients, providing a beautiful, serene, and uplifting environment that aids in healing.

Conclusion

Healing gardens, through their thoughtful design and connection to nature, offer an invaluable respite in a busy world. These gardens across the globe stand as a testament to the positive impact such spaces can have on human health and well-being. They offer a place of peace, healing, and reflection, fostering not just physical, but emotional and psychological healing.

By looking at these successful projects, it becomes evident that a healing garden goes beyond just a well-manicured space; it is a thoughtfully crafted environment, where every element is designed to foster healing. Whether through the sound of water, the scent of flowers, or the sight of lush greenery, these gardens offer a multi-sensory experience that invites individuals to reconnect with nature, offering a healing touch to both mind and body.

the natural lighting in the space. Incorporating elements like lamps with soft lighting can foster a warm and well

The layout should facilitate both social interactions and solitary reflections. Create areas that encourage conversation, and also secluded spots for individuals to have a moment of solitude, fostering a holistic healing environment.

Incorporate elements of nature in the furniture selection process. Consider furniture pieces that have floral or botanical prints or those that incorporate natural elements in their design. This fosters a connection to nature, enhancing the healing process.

Remember to include greenery in the space. Having indoor plants can not only enhance the aesthetic appeal but also contribute to creating a vibrant and nurturing environment. Place plants in strategic locations to create a visually pleasing and balanced layout.

Prioritize accessibility and inclusivity while arranging the furniture. Ensure that the space caters to individuals with different needs, including those with mobility challenges, creating a space where everyone feels welcome and supported.

To sum up, creating a harmonious and healing space involves a careful selection of furniture and a well-planned layout that fosters an optimum healing atmosphere. Incorporating elements that evoke comfort, tranquility, and a connection to nature can greatly enhance the healing properties of the space. The goal is to create an environment that nurtures well-being, encourages relaxation, and fosters a sense of peace and harmony. Through a thoughtful approach to furniture selection and space arrangement, one can create a healing space that serves as a sanctuary of comfort and tranquility.

In addition to the calming influences of blue and green, there is also the potential to use neutral tones like whites, creams, and grays to create a blank canvas that promotes mental clarity and peace. Such tones can evoke a sense of spaciousness, purity, and tranquility, essentially providing a backdrop that doesn't compete for attention, hence allowing other elements in the room to stand out.

Furthermore, the inclusion of biophilic design elements, which focus on human's innate connection to nature, can be remarkably beneficial. Incorporating natural materials, such as wood and stone, can echo the outdoors and provide a grounding, calming influence. Implementing elements like water features can add to the soothing ambiance, the sound of flowing water can offer a serene auditory experience which aids in relaxation and mental rejuvenation.

Color psychology can also play a role in art selections for the space. Art pieces that feature soft, rounded shapes can be soothing, while those with sharp, angular lines might evoke more tension. The choice of artwork should hence be harmonized with the color palette to foster a cohesive and tranquil environment.

When we delve deeper into lighting, we find the concept of layered lighting very prominent. Layered lighting involves using different lighting sources to create a well-rounded lighting solution. It incorporates ambient lighting for overall illumination, task lighting for specific activities, and accent lighting to highlight particular design features or areas in a space.

Moreover, the advancements in technology have led to the advent of smart lighting solutions that can be customized to individual needs, even to the extent of changing the color temperatures as per one's mood or the time of the day, offering a personalized healing space.

Similarly, incorporating daylight harvesting systems can be a wise move. Such systems use sensors to balance the amount of artificial and natural light in a space, promoting energy efficiency while ensuring optimal lighting conditions, and keeping the connection to the natural diurnal cycles intact.

It's also crucial to consider the different needs of various populations. For instance, older individuals might benefit from higher levels of lighting to aid visibility, while children might find softer, diffuse lighting more comforting.

Therefore, a deep understanding and intelligent application of the principles of color and lighting can help in crafting spaces that not only heal but nourish the soul, offering respite and nurturing well-being at multiple levels — a haven where mind, body, and spirit can rejuvenate harmoniously, in synergy with the comforting embrace of thoughtful design.

May need to review the above, possibly duplication of Zen garden material perhaps need to condense some of it to make it more readable

Chapter 5: Commentary on Medical Ethics,

Analyzing the role of the Zen, and shaping medical ethics, providing a fresh perspective to navigate more dilemmas in healthcare

In overview of medical ethics, history, and development

The origins of medical ethics can be traced back to ancient civilizations where medical practitioners were expected to adhere to certain moral guidelines. In ancient Egypt, the Edwin Smith Papyrus outlined early principles guiding medical practices. However, the most noteworthy ancient directive would be the Hippocratic Oath, a pledge attributed to the ancient Greek physician Hippocrates, which laid down several ethical guidelines and principles for the medical fraternity.

As we move into the Middle Ages, the Islamic Golden Age brought about a renaissance in medical ethics, with scholars like Avicenna and Razi contributing substantially by writing extensive texts on ethical medical practices. The modern era witnessed a more structured and institutional approach to medical ethics, with the establishment of ethical committees and organizations devoted to overseeing medical ethics, such as the World Medical Association in 1947.

Today, medical ethics is governed by four principal pillars, which are autonomy, beneficence, non-maleficence, and justice. Autonomy pertains to the respect for individual rights and the freedom to make informed decisions about one's health. Beneficence directs healthcare professionals to act in the best interest of the patient, promoting goodness and well-being.

Non-maleficence, on the other hand, is rooted in the principle of "not harm", advising healthcare providers to avoid actions that could cause harm to patients. Lastly, justice involves treating all patients fairly and equitably, without any form of discrimination.

In the sphere of medical ethics, several stakeholders play crucial roles. Firstly, healthcare practitioners are at the forefront, obligated to adhere to ethical principles in their practice. Then we have patients, who are not just recipients of care but active participants with rights and responsibilities.

In addition, policymakers and legislators have a role to play in shaping the ethical landscape through regulations and policies that guide medical practices. Lastly, society at large is a stakeholder, as medical ethics impacts the broader societal values, norms, and overall health.

Educational institutions and professional bodies also play a pivotal role, as they are responsible for instilling ethical principles in medical students and professionals through training and guidelines.

Conclusion

Medical ethics remains a vibrant and evolving field, constantly adapting to new challenges and developments in the medical field. From ancient guidelines to modern principles and stakeholders encompassing not just healthcare professionals but also patients and society, the realm of medical ethics is an essential pillar in the provision of healthcare, safeguarding moral values and principles, and promoting a humane approach to medicine. It calls for a continuous dialogue and education to ensure the upholding of the highest standards of ethical conduct in the medical profession.

Core Principles of Medical Ethics

Medical ethics stands as an essential guide in the practice of medicine, guiding healthcare professionals to uphold moral principles and values while providing care. In this segment, we will explore the core principles that serve as the bedrock of medical ethics, shedding light on their origins and how they function in today's medical landscape.

As we navigate the evolving pathways of healthcare, the core principles of medical ethics remain our guiding light, ensuring a practice rooted in respect, compassion, and fairness. These principles, deeply ingrained in history and adapted for the modern era, engage a myriad of stakeholders in a collaborative effort to uphold the sanctity of life and the dignity of every individual. Thus, it is incumbent upon us to foster a continual dialogue and education revolving around these principles, embracing the nobility and humanity intrinsic to the field of medicine.

Principles and Ethical Decision-Making: A New Perspective on Ethical Dilemmas as Applied to Medical Ethics

In the dynamic field of healthcare, medical practitioners are frequently met with situations that require sound ethical decision-making based on established principles of medical ethics. In this overview, we will delve into the contemporary approach to ethical dilemmas, focusing on how the principles of medical ethics guide decision-making processes.

The inclusion of Zen principles in medical ethics

Tracing the intersection of Zen philosophy and ethical considerations takes us through a rich history of introspective analysis and a profound understanding of the human condition. Zen, with its roots in Buddhist philosophy, emphasizes mindfulness, compassion, and a deep connection with the present moment. When brought into the dialogue with medical ethics, a tapestry of holistic and mindful approaches to ethical dilemmas begins to unfold, offering a fresh avenue of understanding and resolution that is steeped in centuries-old wisdom.

As the field of medical ethics blossomed, incorporating diverse philosophical viewpoints became vital, bringing Zen into the fold as a tranquil yet powerful advisor in the art of ethical decision-making.

In the present landscape, the core principles of medical ethics find a serene and introspective ally in Zen philosophy. Applying a Zen lens to autonomy encourages a deep, mindful understanding of individual perspectives, fostering a sacred space where patients are empowered to make informed decisions from a place of tranquility and understanding.

Beneficence through a Zen perspective emboldens a practice rooted in compassionate action, with healthcare practitioners embodying a nurturing and healing presence. Non-maleficence takes on a gentle, nurturing persona, guiding practitioners to undertake actions that are in harmony with the principle of "not harm", encouraging a soft, yet firm adherence to protective care.

Justice, viewed through a Zen lens, calls for a harmonious balance, a practice of equitable care that respects the intrinsic dignity and interconnectedness of all beings, promoting an environment of equality and fairness that is mindful of the deeper currents of societal dynamics.

In this enriching confluence of Zen and ethical deliberations, a spectrum of stakeholders come into a harmonious dialogue. Healthcare practitioners find themselves embarking on a journey of self-awareness and mindfulness, fostering a practice grounded in the tranquil strength of Zen principles.

Patients, too, find a voice in this setting, a voice that is encouraged to speak from a place of deep inner wisdom, guided by introspective clarity. Regulatory bodies and ethical committees find in Zen a wise and serene guide, offering paths of resolution that are infused with ancient wisdom and a deep understanding of human nature.

Furthermore, educational institutions stand as nurturing grounds where the seeds of Zen philosophy are sown, encouraging budding practitioners to embrace a path of compassionate and mindful practice.

In the rich and contemplative landscape of Zen philosophy, we find a gentle yet powerful guide in navigating the complex terrain of ethical dilemmas in everyday medical practice. Through the lens of Zen, the principles of medical ethics are viewed with a depth of understanding that embraces the full spectrum of human experience, nurturing a practice that is grounded in compassion, mindfulness, and a harmonious balance with the present moment.

As we embrace the Zen in everyday episode choices, we open ourselves to a deeper understanding and a tranquil strength, forging paths of ethical decision-making that are imbued with wisdom, compassion, and a nurturing embrace of the intrinsic sanctity of all life. It calls us to a practice of gentle yet firm resolve, guiding us to navigate the intricacies of ethical dilemmas with a heart rooted in compassion and a mind anchored in the tranquil depths of mindful presence.

Lessons to Learn from a Zen Perspective: The Role of Mindfulness and Ethical Practices in Mindful Decision-Making

Within the rich philosophical grounds of Zen, there lies an approach to mindful decision-making that integrates a deep awareness and contemplative insight into the fabric of ethical practices, especially pertinent in the realm of medical ethics. This detailed exploration delves into the integration and actualization of Zen principles in daily ethical choices and practices.

From its foundations in Buddhist teachings, the Zen philosophy has always been a vessel carrying the tenets of mindfulness, fostering a space of inner serenity, harmonious interaction, and deep connectivity with the present moment. Historically, this philosophical approach has harmonized perfectly with the evolving journey of medical ethics, gradually fostering a more introspective, balanced, and respectful ethos in medical practices. The development of a mindful ethical framework is seen as a progressive merge of ancient wisdom with modern understanding, grounding decisions in deep reflection and conscious awareness.

Navigating the current healthcare environment through the lens of Zen mindfulness unveils a path where the foundational principles of medical ethics are touched with a deeper sense of awareness and respect for the intricacy of life experiences. Here, autonomy is not just a patient's right to choose but a sacred space of empowered decision-making, rooted in a deep awareness of one's true nature and circumstances.

Beneficence blossoms into a practice of loving-kindness, where actions undertaken are not just for the physical well-being of patients but also to attend to their emotional and spiritual tranquility. Non-maleficence, viewed through the Zen perspective, evolves to signify a commitment to avoiding actions that disrupt the harmonic balance of life, nurturing a protective and respectful attitude towards all life processes.

Justice, in this mindful paradigm, transcends mere fairness to embody a harmonious rhythm of existence, ensuring that each individual is met with understanding, respect, and a genuine effort to understand their unique standpoint in the interconnected web of life.

At this juncture where Zen philosophy meets medical ethics, we find a richer and deeper engagement of all stakeholders in the healthcare spectrum. Healthcare professionals are envisioned as not just healers but as guides assisting individuals in navigating their health journeys with awareness and understanding.

Patients become active participants, bringing to the table a deeply personal insight and a readiness to engage with their health circumstances from a place of conscious choice. Governing bodies, policymakers, and educational institutions are seen as nurturers of this sacred space, fostering a culture of mindfulness that permeates every aspect of healthcare, from policymaking to daily practices.

As we stand on the cusp of a healthcare era steeped in mindfulness and grounded in Zen philosophy, we are called upon to embrace a more holistic, aware, and compassionate approach to ethical practices and decision-making. The Zen perspective invites us to delve deeper, to understand the undercurrents of situations, and to approach dilemmas with a heart open to the subtle nuances of human experience.

Incorporating the teachings of Zen brings forth an enriched space of medical practice where mindfulness is not just a tool but a guiding philosophy, steering the community towards a healthcare paradigm that honors the depth of human experiences. Through this lens, we are encouraged to foster a healthcare system that is both deeply compassionate and wisely aware, moving forward with respect for the interconnectedness of all beings and a commitment to nurturing harmony and balance in every aspect of healthcare. It is a call for a deep, nurturing, and harmonic approach that honors both the individual and the collective, laying down a path of healthcare grounded in understanding, empathy, and a deep respect for the intricate dance of life.

In the modern context, the healthcare sector is increasingly resonating with the power and potential of mindfulness as a tool for diminishing biases. A Zen-focused approach inspires clinicians and healthcare providers to perceive patients holistically, transcending the confines of symptoms and embracing the individual's comprehensive experience, thereby facilitating a gradual reduction in biases.

Renowned practitioners and thinkers, including Thich Nhat Hanh, have fervently advocated for a more profound engagement with mindfulness, a path that naturally culminates in empathy and a grounded understanding, thereby dismantling bias barriers and inviting a holistic perspective in healthcare.

As this discourse unfolds, a multitude of stakeholders find themselves drawn into the enriched narrative. Medical practitioners are progressively aligning with Zen principles, fostering an environment of understanding that surpasses judgment. Patients find themselves in a more receptive and respected space, where they are perceived beyond the apparent symptoms, enhancing a healthcare ethos rooted in mutual respect and empathy.

Simultaneously, ethical boards and governing bodies are playing a cardinal role, sculpting policies and guidelines to advocate a mindful, Zen-inspired approach in healthcare, a transformation enriched by philosophical insights from masters steeped in the wisdom of Zen and mindfulness traditions.

Future Directions

As we steer towards the future, envisioning a framework of medical ethics ingrained with Zen teachings brings forth a landscape where biases are consciously acknowledged and transcended through reflective and mindful practices. The healthcare horizon, as anticipated by experts, embodies deep understanding, compassion, and freedom from preconceived notions and judgments.

Educational realms too are undergoing a transformation, envisaging curricula that embrace Zen philosophies and mindfulness as central tenets, nurturing a forthcoming generation of healthcare professionals who are deeply grounded in the virtues of understanding and empathy, thereby laying the cornerstone for a bias-free healthcare environment.

Moreover, a surge in research elucidating the remarkable implications of mindfulness in healthcare is foreseen, promising a wealth of evidence-backed insights that champion the infusion of Zen principles in daily medical endeavors.

At this critical juncture, where we stand witness to the blossoming relationship between Zen philosophies and medical ethics, we envision a future rich with promise and transformation. Scholarly voices converge on the consensus that embracing a Zen outlook in medical ethics paves the way for a conscientious and cultivated practice of mindfulness, nurturing a healthcare landscape deeply rooted in empathy, understanding, and a genuine reverence for the diverse experiences of every individual.

As we tread forward, the roadmap unfurls as one of enlightened evolution, each step mindful, each decision reflecting a deep-seated commitment to sidestepping biases through the intimate embrace of Zen philosophies. This pathway beckons a healthcare system that reveres empathy and justice, providing a nurturing ground that is not just devoid of biases but transcends them, fostering a sphere of mutual respect and profound understanding, guided by the harmonious, balanced philosophy of Zen mindfulness. It invites us to envision a healthcare sphere where biases are not merely avoided but are transcended, leading to a nurturing space of harmonious, respectful, and deeply understanding engagement

Chapter 6: Intuition in the Art of Diagnosis.

Delving into the mysterious world of clinical intuition, guided by Zen principles to enhance diagnostic accuracy and patient care.

Navigating the intricate pathway of clinical intuition requires a deep, discerning gaze into the somewhat enigmatic arena where instinct meets expertise. Drawing from the wide canvas of Zen teachings, this discussion seeks to elucidate the profound role Zen-guided clinical intuition plays in the rich tapestry of medical ethics and practice, while also underlining its importance.

As we navigate the present landscape, we witness a growing acknowledgment of the role of clinical intuition in the medical realm. Practitioners today are increasingly receptive to the subtle cues and underlying narratives that each patient presents, recognizing the importance of intuitive insights in offering holistic healthcare.

Pioneers in mindfulness, such as Thich Nhat Hanh, have advocated for a practice rooted in deep awareness and connectivity with the present moment, fostering a space where clinical intuition can thrive, guided by a foundation of Zen principles that encourage an empathetic, understanding, and insightful approach to patient care.

Today's medical ecosystem finds various stakeholders dynamically interacting in a space enriched by Zen principles. Medical professionals are evolving, learning to trust their intuitive insights alongside their clinical knowledge, thereby fostering a richer, more nuanced approach to patient care.

Patients find themselves in a nurturing environment where their stories are heard and understood beyond the symptomatic narrative, fostering a deeper connection and a more personalized healthcare experience. Meanwhile, regulatory bodies and ethical committees find themselves in a position to nurture this integration of Zen wisdom and clinical intuition, steering policies and educational directives towards a more intuitive, empathetic, and grounded approach to healthcare.

Looking ahead, we see a trajectory rich in possibilities, with clinical intuition guided by Zen principles carving a space of deep understanding and empathy in the healthcare sector. This approach invites a future where education nurtures intuitive understanding alongside clinical expertise, offering a well-rounded, holistic training ground for future practitioners.

Furthermore, the forefront of research is expected to explore the untapped potentials of clinical intuition further, bringing to light evidence-based insights that validate the importance of intuitive practice in healthcare, grounded in Zen teachings that encourage a mindful, attentive, and deeply connected approach to understanding the intricate narratives of patients.

At this juncture of integration and reflection, we stand on the brink of a transformative journey in healthcare, guided by the profound teachings of Zen. It is a path that recognizes and respects the mysterious role of clinical intuition, understanding its critical place in medical practice.

As we foster a future guided by Zen principles, we open ourselves to the richness of intuitive practice, nurturing a healthcare landscape rooted in deep empathy, understanding, and a harmonious blend of expertise and intuition. It beckons a healthcare scenario where clinicians are not just professionals but intuitive healers, guided by a Zen-inspired vision that recognizes the deep interconnectedness of all beings and the rich tapestry of individual narratives, offering a pathway to healthcare that is both intuitive and enlightened, grounded in the rich philosophical groundings of Zen.

Embarking on the journey to understand the science of intuition and its pivotal role in the enhancement of medical practice necessitates a deep, nuanced examination of how intuitive thought processes can be cultivated and harnessed in healthcare settings. Drawing upon the philosophical underpinnings derived from earlier discussions on Zen principles, we delve into a discourse aimed at understanding and developing intuition in the medical realm.

Retracing the historical footsteps leads us to acknowledge that the concept of intuition has been revered in various philosophical doctrines and scientific explorations, including the profound teachings of Zen Buddhism. Over time, there has been a growing recognition of the well of intuitive knowledge that resides within individuals, encouraging a deep-seated, instinctive understanding of complex realities.

Historically, philosophical maestros, including notable figures such as Carl Jung, have acknowledged the role of intuition as a pillar of human cognition, paving the way for a medical practice that values intuitive insights, fostering an approach rooted in depth, understanding, and an organic connectivity with the nuanced narratives of individual experiences.

As we survey the current medical landscape, we find a burgeoning appreciation for the role of intuition in enhancing healthcare delivery. The modern practitioner is becoming increasingly adept at utilizing intuitive understanding, grounded in a confluence of experience, expertise, and an innate ability to connect deeply with patients, recognizing the multi-dimensional narratives that unfold in each healthcare interaction.

In this setting, inspiration is drawn from leaders in mindfulness, who champion an approach grounded in attentiveness, compassion, and a deep-seated understanding of the human condition, promoting a healthcare approach where intuition is cultivated through sustained practices of mindfulness and conscious presence.

Medical professionals, progressively aligning with a mindset that values intuitive insights, are learning to merge empirical knowledge with intuitive understanding, fostering a practice enriched with depth and nuance.

Patients, too, find themselves in a space where their narratives are embraced with a deeper understanding, facilitating a healthcare journey characterized by empathy and intuitive connectivity. Meanwhile, regulatory bodies and educational institutions have begun to recognize the value of developing intuition, steering the conversation towards a holistic approach to medical education that nurtures both scientific acumen and intuitive understanding.

Looking forward, we envision a healthcare landscape where the science of intuition is central to medical practice. The forthcoming era anticipates an educational paradigm that fosters the cultivation of intuition, developing practitioners who are attuned to the subtle nuances of the human condition and can navigate the complex medical landscape with a fine balance of expertise and intuitive understanding.

As we journey forward, there is an expectation of burgeoning research exploring the science behind intuition, bringing to light evidence-based pathways to cultivate and harness this intrinsic human faculty in medical practice, guided by a philosophy that embraces a harmonious confluence of science and intuition.

As we stand on the cusp of a transformative epoch in healthcare, we embrace the rich potential of intuitive practice guided by the philosophical echoes of Zen teachings. The path unfurls inviting an approach where the science of intuition is revered, fostering a medical landscape characterized by deep empathy, understanding, and a seamless blend of expertise and intuitive insight.

As we navigate this promising trajectory, the vision is one of a healthcare realm grounded in a rich synthesis of scientific knowledge and intuitive understanding, crafting a future where medical practitioners are not only experts in their field but also intuitive healers, capable of navigating the intricate narratives of healthcare with a deep, inherent understanding, rooted in the science of intuition.

Developing Intuitive Skills: A Guide for Physicians on Exercises and Practices

Navigating the complex yet enriching path of developing intuitive skills in the medical field calls for an in-depth exploration of exercises and practices that can hone a physician's ability to understand and interpret situations beyond just the empirical data. As we unravel this vital aspect, we delve deep into understanding how the nurturing of intuitive skills can become a cornerstone in a physician's practice.

To comprehend the genesis of intuitive skills, we steer our gaze towards historical delineations where intuition was seen as a potent force guiding individuals in various professions, including medical practitioners. Through historical epochs, there have been physician pioneers who have leaned on their intuitive understanding to unravel complex medical cases, setting a precedent for a practice rich in intuitive insights and grounded in deep connectivity with the self and the patients.

Fast forward to today's dynamic healthcare landscape; we witness a growing recognition and emphasis on developing intuitive skills. Physicians now have access to a myriad of exercises and practices, fostering a deeper connection with their intuitive selves. The contemporaneous medical environment promotes mindfulness, reflective practices, and guided imagery exercises as potent tools to nurture and develop intuitive faculties, thereby aiding in a more empathetic and insightful practice.

At the nexus of this evolving dialogue stand a multitude of stakeholders — physicians, psychologists, and even patients who are actively involved in fostering a space where intuition is respected and nurtured. Physicians are gradually embracing exercises like mindful meditation and reflective journaling to hone their intuitive skills, weaving them into their daily routines to foster a practice grounded in intuitive understanding and empathetic connectivity.

Future Directions

Peering into the potential future landscapes, we envisage a medical realm where intuitive skills are central to physician training and practice. The foreseeability extends to medical curricula incorporating modules and workshops dedicated to nurturing intuitive skills through a variety of exercises and practices. Moreover, it anticipates a research-led foray into understanding the science behind intuition, encouraging a practice grounded in evidence-based intuitive methodologies, offering a rich blend of scientific knowledge and intuitive insight.

As we stand at this juncture, rich with potential and promise, we acknowledge the transformative role that developing intuitive skills can play in the broader spectrum of medical ethics and practice. The trajectory suggests a harmonious blend of science and intuition, fostering a generation of physicians adept in marrying empirical knowledge with intuitive insight.

As we foster a future where intuitive skills are not just an addendum but a vital aspect of medical practice, we anticipate a realm where physicians are equipped with a rich repertoire of exercises and practices to nurture their intuitive faculties. Thus, ushering in an era where healthcare is not just science-driven but intuitively guided, offering a deeply empathetic, understanding, and enriched patient care experience, grounded in the nurturing of intuitive skills.

Developing intuitive skills in the medical practice remains a pivotal focus, bringing together historical insights and present advancements facilitated by expert advice. The harmonization of intuitive and empirical approaches can essentially enhance the holistic approach to patient care.

History and Development

Drawing from the wellspring of history, we find a mosaic of instances where medical practitioners have leveraged their intuitive faculties to reach diagnoses that were not immediately apparent through conventional methods. The annals of medical history are punctuated with stories of doctors who, guided by a hunch, pursued lines of treatment that eventually led to recovery, thereby affirming the valuable role that intuition plays in medical diagnostics and treatment.

Present Day

As we navigate the currents of present-day medical practice, we find an increasing number of physicians endorsing the incorporation of intuitive thinking in their daily routines. Many have narrated instances where a sudden insight or a gut feeling led them to explore alternative diagnostic paths, often resulting in more accurate diagnoses and personalized treatments. These narratives form a compelling tapestry of evidence in favor of nurturing intuition, as practitioners recount moments where their intuitive skills proved to be a linchpin in facilitating successful outcomes.

The discourse on the role of intuition in medical practice is enriched by the contribution of a diverse group of stakeholders encompassing physicians, medical researchers, and patients. Today's healthcare landscape is populated with stories of patients who have benefited immensely from a physician's intuitive insight, painting a canvas rich with instances where intuitive thinking facilitated recovery pathways that were both unexpected and revolutionary. Medical researchers too add to this narrative, delving into the underlying mechanisms that drive intuitive thinking, thus adding a layer of scientific validation to these experiences.

Future Directions

Looking ahead, we stand on the threshold of exciting possibilities. The momentum gained from the success stories of today promises to shape a future where training in intuitive skills is a cornerstone in the education of medical practitioners. The medical fraternity is abuzz with anticipation, envisioning a future steeped in a balanced approach that harmoniously blends intuitive thinking with scientific rigor, thus opening up pathways to innovative and patient-centric solutions.

As we take stock of the compelling narratives and the success stories that mark the journey of intuition in medical practice, we find ourselves amidst a revolution of sorts. The rich repertoire of case studies paints a vivid picture of a healthcare landscape where intuition and science walk hand in hand. It tells a story of a future where the fostering of intuitive skills not only complements scientific understanding but elevates it, bringing to the fore a medical practice that is both intuitive and evidence-based, thus promising a future where healthcare is more personalized, compassionate, and effective. It is a journey of discovering the immense potential that lies in harmonizing intuition with science, guided by the beacon of success stories from the past and present, illuminating the pathway to a brighter, more intuitive future in healthcare.

Finding the Middle Ground: Balancing Intuition and Evidence-Based Medicine

As we traverse the evolving landscape of healthcare, we find ourselves in the midst of an important dialogue – seeking the equilibrium where intuition harmoniously coexists with evidence-based medicine, a confluence that promises a more rounded approach to patient care.

Historically, the practice of medicine has swung between reliance on intuitive judgments and strict adherence to evidence-based protocols. Delving into the annals of medical history, we find a rich tapestry of narratives where seasoned physicians relied heavily on their intuitive insights, often successfully diagnosing conditions that eluded conventional diagnostic paradigms. This journey through time offers us a glimpse of the potential harbored in a practice that judiciously balances intuition with evidence, offering a rich ground to foster a medical practice that draws from the best of both worlds.

In the contemporary medical landscape, there is a burgeoning recognition of the value in marrying intuition with evidence-based practice. Physicians and medical practitioners recount experiences where listening to their intuitive nudges and complementing them with scientific evidence facilitated more accurate diagnoses and treatment paths. This synergistic approach is emerging as a potent tool, fostering a healthcare environment that is both scientifically grounded and intuitively guided, promising a rich space for nuanced patient care.

Today, a broad spectrum of individuals, including practitioners, academics, and patients, are actively engaged in shaping this narrative. The stories emerging from various quarters echo a collective aspiration to forge a practice that honors both the intuitive whispers and the empirical evidence, creating a collaborative and empathetic healthcare space. Medical scholars and practitioners alike are delving into research, seeking to understand the intrinsic connections between intuitive reasoning and evidence-based practice, thus adding depth to this ongoing dialogue.

Future Directions

As we peer into the future of healthcare, we envision a vibrant landscape where training modules are designed to foster a balanced approach, nurturing the capacity to fluidly navigate between intuition and evidence. This vision of the future foresees educational paradigms that encourage budding practitioners to develop intuitive skills while maintaining a strong foundation in evidence-based practice. The horizon is ripe with potential, promising a healthcare system that values the contribution of both intuitive insights and scientific rigor, paving the way for a harmonized approach to medical practice.

As we stand at this promising junction, it is clear that the path forward is one of integration, where intuition and evidence-based medicine collaboratively shape a more empathetic and effective healthcare system. The rich narratives and extensive discussions in the field underscore a unanimous aspiration for a future where medical practice is a symphony of intuitive understanding and scientific evidence, operating in harmony to offer a healthcare experience that is deeply sensitive, insightful, and grounded in empirical reality. It beckons a new era in healthcare, one that honors the deep-seated intuitive capabilities of practitioners while revering the sanctity of scientific evidence, thus crafting a future that is both compassionate and scientifically robust. It is a vision of healthcare that stands as a testament to the incredible potential that lies in finding the middle ground, promising a journey toward a more balanced, insightful, and holistic approach to medicine.

Chapter 7: Zen and End-of-Life Care

Exploring the sensitive topic of end-of-life care to the length of Zen, promoting peace and understanding in the final stages of life.

As we approach the delicate and profound topic of end-of-life care, it becomes imperative to further cultivate a practice that not only leans on empirical evidence but also embraces the intuitive, holistic approach inspired by Zen philosophy. This philosophy, which promotes peace, understanding, and a deep connection to the present moment, can serve as a valuable guide in navigating the intricate landscape of end-of-life care. Here we venture to explore the convergence of intuition and evidence-based medicine in this context, envisioning a practice grounded in compassion and understanding.

Historical Context

Historically, end-of-life care has navigated the tender ground of human existence, a space where scientific interventions often meet their limits, necessitating a compassionate, intuitive approach. The teachings of Zen, which emphasize the importance of being fully present and embracing the transient nature of life, offer a rich resource for fostering a caring approach deeply rooted in empathy and understanding. Zen's contemplative principles could potentially enhance the medical fraternity's ability to provide care that is grounded in both empirical evidence and intuitive understanding.

In the current discourse on end-of-life care, there is a budding recognition of the value that Zen philosophy can bring in fostering a peaceful, understanding environment during the final stages of life. Medical practitioners are increasingly becoming aware of the limitations of a purely evidence-based approach in this delicate stage. Zen, with its emphasis on harmony, peace, and living in the moment, offers a pathway to navigate this time with grace, encouraging an approach that listens intuitively to the needs and wishes of the patient, promoting peace and understanding through an inherently compassionate lens.

Engagement in this compassionate approach to end-of-life care is a multifaceted endeavor involving healthcare professionals, caregivers, patients, and their families. A wide array of stakeholders, including those rooted in spiritual and philosophical communities, are coming forward to champion the integration of Zen principles in healthcare settings, fostering spaces where deep understanding and empathy are at the forefront, thus enabling a gentle transition during the end stages of life.

Future Directions

Looking forward to the future, it seems promising to envision training programs incorporating Zen philosophy to foster an intuitive, empathetic approach alongside evidence-based protocols. By facilitating a deep understanding of the principles of Zen, which include meditation and mindfulness, future healthcare practitioners could be empowered to offer end-of-life care that is both scientifically grounded and spiritually nurturing, promoting peace and understanding in the final stages of life.

As we delve deeper into the exploration of this sensitive subject, a harmonized approach that integrates the Zen philosophy with evidence-based medicine emerges as a pathway filled with hope and potential. The interweaving of the calming Zen perspectives with medical expertise promises a healthcare scenario where end-of-life care is not just about managing symptoms but about promoting peace, understanding, and a serene acceptance of life's transience. By fostering a practice that draws from the rich teachings of Zen, a door opens to a kinder, more compassionate end-of-life care that honors both the empirical and the intuitive, guiding individuals to a peaceful transition that respects the sanctity of life in all its phases.

Exploring the Middle Ground in End-of-Life Care: A Zen Perspective

As we approach the delicate and profound topic of end-of-life care, it becomes imperative to further cultivate a practice that not only leans on empirical evidence but also embraces the intuitive, holistic approach inspired by Zen philosophy. This philosophy, which promotes peace, understanding, and a deep connection to the present moment, can serve as a valuable guide in navigating the intricate landscape of end-of-life care. Here we venture to explore the convergence of intuition and evidence-based medicine in this context, envisioning a practice grounded in compassion and understanding.

Historical Context

Historically, end-of-life care has navigated the tender ground of human existence, a space where scientific interventions often meet their limits, necessitating a compassionate, intuitive approach. The teachings of Zen, which emphasize the importance of being fully present and embracing the transient nature of life, offer a rich resource for fostering a caring approach deeply rooted in empathy and understanding. Zen's contemplative principles could potentially enhance the medical fraternity's ability to provide care that is grounded in both empirical evidence and intuitive understanding.

In the current discourse on end-of-life care, there is a budding recognition of the value that Zen philosophy can bring in fostering a peaceful, understanding environment during the final stages of life. Medical practitioners are increasingly becoming aware of the limitations of a purely evidence-based approach in this delicate stage. Zen, with its emphasis on harmony, peace, and living in the moment, offers a pathway to navigate this time with grace, encouraging an approach that listens intuitively to the needs and wishes of the patient, promoting peace and understanding through an inherently compassionate lens.

Engagement in this compassionate approach to end-of-life care is a multifaceted endeavor involving healthcare professionals, caregivers, patients, and their families. A wide array of stakeholders, including those rooted in spiritual and philosophical communities, are coming forward to champion the integration of Zen principles in healthcare settings, fostering spaces where deep understanding and empathy are at the forefront, thus enabling a gentle transition during the end stages of life.

Future Directions

Looking forward to the future, it seems promising to envision training programs incorporating Zen philosophy to foster an intuitive, empathetic approach alongside evidence-based protocols. By facilitating a deep understanding of the principles of Zen, which include meditation and mindfulness, future healthcare practitioners could be empowered to offer end-of-life care that is both scientifically grounded and spiritually nurturing, promoting peace and understanding in the final stages of life.

At present, a diverse group of concerned, individuals including healthcare practitioners, policymakers, families, and patients from varied cultural backgrounds, are coming together to shape a more inclusive discourse on end-of-life care. Scholars and researchers globally are increasingly investigating the cross-cultural dimensions, striving to foster a practice that is both scientifically robust and culturally sensitive.

Looking into the future, it is imperative to develop training curricula for healthcare providers that are inclusive of cross-cultural competencies, aiming to bridge the gap between different cultural understandings and expectations surrounding end-of-life care. This would entail a global collaboration to foster education that is rich in diversity, offering future practitioners a toolkit that is grounded in empirical evidence while being deeply respectful and understanding of different cultural nuances.

As we stand at this juncture, the path forward in understanding the current state of end-of-life care is seemingly leading toward a more inclusive and comprehensive approach. The evolving discourse suggests a promising future where end-of-life care is seen through a global lens, taking into account the rich diversity of cultural perspectives and practices. This convergence of scientific understanding and cross-cultural empathy promises to guide the healthcare system toward offering end-of-life care that is respectful, dignified, and profoundly sensitive to the myriad cultural tapestries that adorn our global society, ushering in a new era of compassionate and individualized care.

In the ever-evolving tapestry of healthcare, one of the most profound aspects we find ourselves discussing is the care and guidance required in the final stages of life. It is a time that calls for a delicate balance between medical expertise and heartfelt understanding, where both the patients and their families' needs and concerns are met with utmost empathy and proficiency.

History and Development

Looking back at the historical approach to end-of-life care, we find a trajectory of ever-deepening understanding and empathy toward the patients and their families. Historically, a considerable emphasis has been placed on alleviating physical pain; however, with time, there has been a growing acknowledgment of the emotional, spiritual, and psychological dimensions that come into play. The journey has been one of gradual enrichment, with a deepening understanding of the need to incorporate a compassionate approach, intertwining medical expertise with a gentle human touch.

In the current healthcare landscape, we witness a progressive trend where end-of-life care encompasses a holistic approach that is both scientifically grounded and intuitively guided. Medical professionals are encouraged to engage their intuitive faculties to foster a space of understanding and empathy, alongside employing evidence-based methods to manage pain and other physical symptoms effectively. Moreover, it's a time when the concerns and needs of the families are given paramount importance, nurturing a support system that stands fortified with understanding, patience, and empathy.

Future Directions

As we envisage the future, we anticipate an even more integrated approach to end-of-life care. Future trajectories hint at personalized care plans developed through a collaborative effort involving the patient, family, and a multidisciplinary team of professionals. This envisioned approach seeks to harmonize intuitive understanding with scientific knowledge, facilitating a journey where the final stages of life are met with dignity, grace, and deep respect for the patient's wishes and the family's concerns.

As we foster a conversation around end-of-life care, it is clear that the path forward is one of compassionate integration, where the physical, emotional, and spiritual needs of patients and families are met with a tender and understanding approach. The rich discussions underline a unanimous aspiration for a future healthcare scenario that is steeped in compassion, where the final stages of life are navigated with a harmonized approach of intuition and evidence-based practices. It is a vision filled with hope and understanding, where the end-of-life journey is treated with the grace it deserves, enveloping patients and families in a canopy of care that is both medically proficient and deeply empathic, paving the way for a dignified, respectful, and peaceful passage.

Navigating the Final Stages of Life: Addressing the Needs and Concerns of Patients and Families

In the ever-evolving tapestry of healthcare, one of the most profound aspects we find ourselves discussing is the care and guidance required in the final stages of life. It is a time that calls for a delicate balance between medical expertise and heartfelt understanding, where both the patients and their families' needs and concerns are met with utmost empathy and proficiency.

Looking back at the historical approach to end-of-life care, we find a trajectory of ever-deepening understanding and empathy toward the patients and their families. Historically, a considerable emphasis has been placed on alleviating physical pain; however, with time, there has been a growing acknowledgment of the emotional, spiritual, and psychological dimensions that come into play. The journey has been one of gradual enrichment, with a deepening understanding of the need to incorporate a compassionate approach, intertwining medical expertise with a gentle human touch.

In the current healthcare landscape, we witness a progressive trend where end-of-life care encompasses a holistic approach that is both scientifically grounded and intuitively guided. Medical professionals are encouraged to engage their intuitive faculties to foster a space of understanding and empathy, alongside employing evidence-based methods to manage pain and other physical symptoms effectively. Moreover, it's a time when the concerns and needs of the families are given paramount importance, nurturing a support system that stands fortified with understanding, patience, and empathy.

There is a concerted effort to bring a rounded perspective that honors the individual's wishes while providing the family with the support and guidance they require, creating a harmonious environment grounded in empathy and understanding.

As we envisage the future, we anticipate an even more integrated approach to end-of-life care. Future trajectories hint at personalized care plans developed through a collaborative effort involving the patient, family, and a multidisciplinary team of professionals. This envisioned approach seeks to harmonize intuitive understanding with scientific knowledge, facilitating a journey where the final stages of life are met with dignity, grace, and deep respect for the patient's wishes and the family's concerns.

As we foster a conversation around end-of-life care, it is clear that the path forward is one of compassionate integration, where the physical, emotional, and spiritual needs of patients and families are met with a tender and understanding approach. The rich discussions underline a unanimous aspiration for a future healthcare scenario that is steeped in compassion, where the final stages of life are navigated with a harmonized approach of intuition and evidence-based practices. It is a vision filled with hope and understanding, where the end-of-life journey is treated with the grace it deserves, enveloping patients and families in a canopy of care that is both medically proficient and deeply empathic, paving the way for a dignified, respectful, and peaceful passage.

Navigating the Final Stages of Life: Zen Teachings on Mortality

In the expansive discourse on healthcare and end-of-life care, Zen teachings offer profound insights into mortality, guiding individuals and their families in navigating the inevitable journey with wisdom, acceptance, and tranquility. It is imperative to delve deep into Zen teachings on mortality to foster an environment of understanding, peace, and compassionate care during the final stages of life.

Zen Buddhism has a rich history of meditative practices and philosophical insights that delve deep into the nature of life and death. Traditionally, Zen teachings emphasize the transient nature of existence, promoting an understanding of mortality grounded in the principles of impermanence and interconnectedness of all life forms. This understanding encourages individuals to live fully in the present moment, embracing the ever-changing flow of life with acceptance and awareness.

In contemporary settings, Zen teachings are gradually being recognized and integrated into end-of-life care, guiding individuals to navigate their mortality with a deep sense of peace and acceptance. This approach encourages a holistic viewpoint, where death is not seen as an end but a transformation, a natural process in the cycle of life and death. Medical professionals are guided to foster a space of compassionate care, understanding the deep-seated fears associated with mortality and helping individuals approach the end-of-life transition with serenity and acceptance.

Caregivers and other concerned individuals work hand in hand with the family members to create a nurturing environment, encouraging open conversations around mortality that are grounded in Zen philosophy, which embraces the transient nature of life. This approach helps in demystifying death, encouraging individuals to face mortality with an open heart and a tranquil mind.

As we look towards the future, there is a vision of deepening the integration of Zen teachings in end-of-life care, emphasizing individualized care plans that embrace the impermanent nature of life. This approach promotes a harmonized care path, fostering a space of peace and acceptance that allows individuals to navigate their mortality with grace and dignity. It advocates for a heightened consciousness, where individuals, guided by Zen teachings, can experience a transition marked with tranquility and a deep understanding of the interconnectedness of life and death.

In conclusion, Zen teachings offer a profound and nurturing approach to navigating mortality, emphasizing the transient nature of life and fostering an environment of acceptance and peace. Integrating Zen philosophies into end-of-life care encourages individuals to approach death with a calm mind and a heart full of acceptance. It helps in fostering a serene end-of-life journey, characterized by deep mindfulness, tranquility, and a profound understanding of the cyclical nature of life and death. Thus, Zen teachings guide us in creating a compassionate and understanding approach to mortality, offering a path of grace, dignity, and serenity in the final stages of life, where individuals and families learn to embrace the transient nature of existence with peace and harmony.

Navigating the Final Stages of Life: Applying Zen Principles in End-of-Life Scenarios

As we continue to foster deeper understanding and compassionate approaches in end-of-life scenarios, applying Zen principles emerges as a profound pathway to guide individuals and their families through this pivotal journey. Incorporating the wisdom encapsulated in Zen teachings can significantly transform the experiences of individuals navigating the end of life, enveloping them in an ambiance of peace, acceptance, and mindful presence.

Tracing the roots of Zen Buddhism, we find a rich tradition focusing on meditation, mindfulness, and the understanding of the impermanent nature of life. These foundational principles have guided individuals in facing mortality with a calm and accepting demeanor, nurturing a profound connection with the present moment. Over the centuries, the integration of Zen principles in end-of-life scenarios has been deepening, focusing on a compassionate and mindful approach towards the dying process, emphasizing presence, acceptance, and the release of fear.

In the current landscape of end-of-life care, Zen principles are being employed more extensively to foster an environment of tranquility, acceptance, and deep connection. These principles advocate for the cultivation of a calm mind and a harmonious approach to the natural cycle of life and death. Healthcare providers are learning to utilize Zen meditation techniques to facilitate peaceful transitions, encouraging patients to embrace the present moment fully, thereby reducing anxiety and fear. Moreover, mindfulness practices guided by Zen teachings are aiding in alleviating physical pain and emotional distress, nurturing a space of peace and acceptance.

The application of Zen principles in end-of-life scenarios invites a collaborative approach, where medical professionals work alongside Zen practitioners, spiritual counselors, and family members to create a nurturing and serene environment. Zen practitioners can offer guided meditation sessions, helping individuals navigate their fears and anxieties with a grounded presence. Furthermore, spiritual counselors are available to offer insights into the Zen philosophies of impermanence and interconnectedness, fostering a deeper understanding and acceptance of the dying process

Looking forward, the application of Zen principles in end-of-life scenarios is envisioned to take a more structured form. The creation of personalized care plans grounded in Zen philosophy can significantly aid in guiding individuals gracefully through the final stages of life. The future holds a promise of training healthcare professionals in Zen meditation techniques, thereby enhancing their ability to offer compassionate care. Moreover, developing spaces that embody the tranquility and peace advocated by Zen principles is seen as a vital step in facilitating serene and dignified end-of-life experiences.

Incorporating Zen principles in end-of-life care forms a pathway laden with tranquility, acceptance, and mindful presence, fostering an environment that recognizes the transient yet beautiful nature of life. These teachings encourage a harmonious transition, where individuals can navigate the complexities of mortality with grace and dignity, grounded in the present moment. The integration of Zen principles encourages individuals and families to embrace the impermanent nature of life, fostering a compassionate and mindful approach to death, and offering a sanctuary of peace, understanding, and grace in the final stages of life. This thoughtful approach promises to reshape end-of-life experiences into journeys of peace, dignity, and profound acceptance, paving a harmonious path for both individuals and their families.

In the pursuit of providing comprehensive care during the final stages of life, creating a peaceful environment stands as a cornerstone in supporting end-of-life patients and their families. Drawing from an enriched understanding of Zen philosophies and present healthcare paradigms, this presentation delves into the strategies and approaches necessary to foster a tranquil environment that aligns with the principles of dignity, compassion, and respect for end-of-life patients.

Historically, the approach to end-of-life care has evolved significantly, progressing from a predominantly medical focus to a more holistic approach that includes spiritual and emotional well-being. In recent times, the understanding and application of creating a peaceful environment have been deeply influenced by Zen teachings, which emphasize the impermanence of life and the importance of being present in the moment. This history serves as a foundation in the evolving narrative to provide end-of-life patients with a tranquil setting that echoes with serenity and understanding.

Today, the endeavor to create a peaceful environment takes a multi-faceted approach. Healthcare facilities are increasingly adopting the principles of Zen philosophy to craft spaces that are calming and soothing. This includes not only physical alterations such as comfortable bedding and serene landscapes but also the integration of meditative practices and mindfulness sessions that guide individuals to maintain a peaceful state of mind. Pain management strategies are being enhanced with techniques derived from Zen practices, aiming to reduce suffering and foster a state of calm and acceptance.

The collaborative efforts to create this peaceful environment bring together a team of healthcare professionals, spiritual guides, Zen practitioners, and family members. Zen practitioners may offer guidance in meditation techniques, helping to foster a mindset of tranquility and acceptance. Meanwhile, spiritual guides assist in navigating the emotional and spiritual concerns that arise, facilitating open dialogues that are grounded in compassion and understanding. The family, too, is guided to maintain a harmonious atmosphere, learning to be present and offering support through a loving and understanding lens.

As we move forward, there is a growing emphasis on personalizing the environment to suit the preferences and needs of the individual. Future strategies envision a comprehensive approach where healthcare settings might include serene meditation rooms, gardens to foster connectivity with nature and personalized rooms where families can spend quality time with their loved ones. Moreover, the development of training programs for healthcare professionals to deepen their understanding of Zen principles is seen as a pivotal step in fostering a truly peaceful environment for end-of-life patients.

To sum up, creating a peaceful environment for end-of-life patients is a nuanced endeavor that draws heavily from the rich philosophical backdrop of Zen teachings and contemporary healthcare insights. It is a journey that prioritizes serenity, understanding, and compassion, encouraging a harmonious transition through the final stages of life. As we forge ahead, the integration of Zen principles with modern healthcare approaches offers a beacon of hope, promising an end-of-life experience characterized by peace, dignity, and deep respect for the transient nature of life, guiding individuals to a graceful passage enveloped in tranquility and love.

Creating a peaceful environment for end-of-life patients indeed goes beyond medical care and touches upon the emotional, spiritual, and psychological facets of the human experience. Delving deeper, we find that space design holds a pivotal role in facilitating an environment that fosters peace, comfort, and serenity during the final stages of life. Let us explore the multi-faceted approach to designing spaces that resonate with tranquility and facilitate a peaceful transition.

Currently, there is a conscientious movement towards integrating aesthetics and therapeutic designs in healthcare settings to foster a harmonious and peaceful environment for end-of-life patients. The focus is on creating spaces that provide a sense of calm, embrace natural elements, and facilitate meditation and reflection.

In conclusion, the role of space design in creating a peaceful environment for end-of-life patients cannot be overstated. It is a multidisciplinary endeavor that seeks to create nurturing spaces that facilitate peaceful and dignified end-of-life experiences. By focusing on elements such as natural integration, personalization, and aesthetic enrichment, we pave the way for spaces that echo with tranquility, comfort, and respect for the individual's journey, fostering a setting that supports both the patients and their families as they navigate this profound phase of life with grace and serenity.

Navigating the Final Stages of Life: Creating a Zen-Inspired End-of-Life Care Routine

In the dynamic landscape of healthcare, a crucial topic that demands careful consideration is curating an end-of-life care routine inspired by Zen principles, which emphasizes peace, presence, and deep connection with oneself and their surroundings. This approach calls for a harmonious amalgamation of meditative wisdom and healthcare expertise, providing a safe space where both the patients and their families can navigate the final stages of life with grace and tranquility. Here we will delve deep into how Zen-inspired principles can be brought to fruition, through thoughtful routines for end-of-life care.

Historically, healthcare has been centered around treating physical ailments, with little consideration for the emotional and spiritual well-being of the individual. However, over time, there has been a gradual inclination towards holistic care, borrowing from ancient Zen principles that focus on the present moment, fostering a deep connection with oneself, and nurturing serenity through simplicity. This philosophical backdrop has influenced the development of an end-of-life care routine that seeks to create a peaceful atmosphere conducive to reflection and tranquility.

In the contemporary healthcare scenario, Zen-inspired end-of-life care routines are gaining prominence, integrating meditative practices, and fostering environments that encourage tranquility and self-awareness. Healthcare providers are considering elements like peaceful surroundings, relaxed breathing techniques, and engaging in mindful conversations to facilitate a sense of calm and presence.

Creating a connection with nature by incorporating elements such as natural lighting, indoor plants, and soothing sounds that mimic natural environments, fosters a calming atmosphere that facilitates mindfulness and reflection.

Encouraging open, honest, and compassionate dialogues, allowing individuals to express their fears, hopes, and desires freely, fostering a space of understanding and empathy.

Integrating daily meditation sessions to help individuals remain centered and find peace through focused breathing and mindful reflection.

Looking towards the future, there is scope for a more personalized Zen-inspired routine, designed keeping in mind the individual preferences and needs of the patients. It could encompass a wide range of services including:

Creating personalized meditation tracks, that cater to the individual's preferences, focusing on themes that bring them peace and tranquility.

Expanding the scope of nature therapy, involving therapeutic garden walks and nature sound therapy to foster a deep connection with the natural elements.

As we forge a path forward, it is evident that a Zen-inspired end-of-life care routine holds the promise of a peaceful and mindful transition through the final stages of life. Drawing from ancient Zen philosophies, it encourages a deep connection with one's inner self and the environment, facilitating a space of tranquility, presence, and grace. As we integrate these principles into healthcare, we venture into a future where end-of-life care is not just about alleviating physical pain but nurturing the soul, providing a compassionate canopy of peace and mindfulness, and fostering a dignified and serene passage.

Navigating the Final Stages of Life: Zen, End-of-Life Care, and Personal Narratives - Lessons Learned

In the evolving field of healthcare, focusing on end-of-life care through the lens of Zen teachings and personal narratives opens a pathway to not just address physical ailments but also to foster a holistic approach that recognizes the intricate weave of life experiences, wisdom, and the profound lessons learned during this stage. Below we will explore the profound connections between Zen teachings, end-of-life care, and the personal narratives which carry invaluable lessons for all involved.

Currently, end-of-life care is witnessing a beautiful blend of Zen teachings that focus on mindfulness, being present, and embracing the transient nature of life, with careful listening to personal narratives, which offers a rich tapestry of the individual's life, their lessons learned, and the wisdom they wish to impart. This has ushered in an era of holistic care that is both deep and profoundly personal, weaving in elements of meditation, conscious presence, and the cherished personal stories that shape the individual's worldview.

Looking forward, we envision an ever-evolving approach which:

Encourages collaborative storytelling sessions where individuals can share their stories, forging connections and mutual understanding through shared experiences.

The integration of regular mindfulness workshops, based on Zen teachings, into the healthcare routine to nurture a space of peace and acceptance.

As we explore the intricate relationship between Zen teachings, end-of-life care, and personal narratives, it becomes evident that a caring approach, embedded in mindfulness and deep respect for personal stories, paves the way for a journey filled with grace, learning, and profound respect. By honoring individual narratives and fostering an environment rooted in Zen principles, the final stages of life become a rich canvas of shared experiences, insights, and cherished moments, nurturing a journey marked with dignity, understanding, and deep connections. It is a path of heartfelt care, where each narrative becomes a beacon of wisdom, guiding others while crafting a peaceful, reflective, and nourished space for the end-of-life journey.

In the ever-evolving field of healthcare, one critical facet that often comes to focus is the role and impact of bereavement care. Bereavement, the period of mourning and grief experienced following the death of a loved one, holds a significant place in the healthcare spectrum. It is a time that demands sensitivity, understanding, and a holistic approach to aid individuals and families in navigating the complex emotions and realities they face. Here we explore the intricate dance between bereavement and healthcare, emphasizing the transformative learnings and approaches that have shaped the current landscape.

At present, the healthcare sector has embraced a more inclusive approach to bereavement, understanding that it is an integral part of the end-of-life care spectrum. The current framework involves:

Offering counseling services and support groups to help individuals navigate their grief journey, providing a space for sharing and mutual understanding.

Provision of resources such as literature, workshops, and seminars that offer guidance and information on coping with loss.

The modern approach to bereavement care is collaborative, involving healthcare providers, counselors, therapists, and support groups working in synergy to offer a supportive network for the bereaved. The role of family and friends is also pivotal, providing a nurturing environment for the individual navigating the loss.

As we cast a gaze towards the future, the path seems to be steering towards an even more personalized and comprehensive approach to bereavement care. Potential developments might include:

Chapter 8: The Future of Zen-Inspired Medicine

Some concluding thoughts

The Harmonious Union: Zen, Modern Medicine, and Timeless Healing Traditions

In the vast realm of healthcare, one might perceive Zen, modern medicine, and age-old alternative practices as distinctive entities. Yet, when we delve deeper, we find they are more than just parallel paths; they are interconnected strands that, when woven together, create a comprehensive tapestry of holistic healing.

Zen introduces us to the "beginner's mind" or shoshin. This unique perspective encourages approaching every experience with a fresh, unbiased view, reminiscent of a child's innocent curiosity. Such an outlook becomes revolutionary in the world of medicine. As medical practitioners engage with diverse patients, each bringing their individual stories and challenges, embracing Shoshin ensures that every case is approached without prejudice, allowing for clearer judgment and more empathetic care.

This philosophy doesn't undermine the importance of accumulated medical knowledge; instead, it emphasizes the harmonious marriage of tried-and-tested wisdom with fresh, present-moment insights.

Architectural Harmony: Zen and Diverse Medical Traditions

Zen isn't just a personal practice. Its philosophy permeates the design and ambiance of spaces, guiding the creation of environments that soothe and heal. Drawing inspiration from Zen, modern therapeutic spaces can be transformed into sanctuaries of calm, marked by minimalist aesthetics and profound connections to nature.

Picture a healthcare facility where walls radiate calm with gentle colors, and where rooms open up to serene gardens or peaceful landscapes. In these spaces, waiting areas become more than holding zones. They evolve into reflective retreats, adorned with Zen gardens, soft natural lighting, and tranquil water features.

Incorporated within such environments could be specialized sections dedicated to alternative healing modalities. Acupuncture chambers influenced by traditional Chinese medicine, consultation rooms for Ayurvedic treatments echoing East Indian wisdom, and tranquil corners for homeopathic discussions could seamlessly blend in, creating an integrative healing experience.

Furthermore, an auditory shift could enhance the therapeutic experience. Replacing the sterile beeps of machines with nature-inspired sounds, such as water flowing or birds chirping, could offer solace to patients and energize healthcare practitioners, fostering an ambiance where both modern and traditional healing methods thrive.

The Confluence of Healing Philosophies

At the heart of Zen is the profound acknowledgment of interconnectedness. This belief aligns seamlessly with the therapeutic world, advocating for a symbiotic relationship between doctor and patient. While modern medicine is armed with cutting-edge technology and research, traditional practices bring with them centuries of holistic insights. When these two worlds merge, patients benefit from a comprehensive care approach, addressing both physiological symptoms and the holistic well-being of the individual.

The Dance of Change and Diverse Healing Modalities

Zen teachings constantly remind us of the impermanence of life. In the realm of health, this translates to recognizing and respecting the ever-evolving nature of our well-being. Modern medicine, with its solutions and interventions, meets its perfect complement in alternative therapies like Chinese medicine, Ayurveda, and homeopathy. These age-old traditions emphasize alignment with nature, seeking harmony and balance rather than just curing symptoms.

In Closing: A Symphony of Healing Arts

This journey highlights the potential richness of healthcare when Zen principles, modern medical practices, and ancient healing traditions converge. Such an approach transforms hospitals and clinics from merely clinical spaces to comprehensive wellness sanctuaries. In these sanctuaries, healthcare practitioners cater to the multi-dimensional needs of patients, addressing the physical, emotional, and spiritual realms. Through the amalgamation of time-tested wisdom, advanced science, and the timeless art of Zen, we pave the way for a harmonious, holistic health journey for all.

The end .. the beginning of a new adventure.

The reader is encouraged to provide feedback. Please share your experiences. Insights suggestions regarding this book.

Thank you so much for your time. I hope you enjoy the experience. Be well always.

Dr Victor Denis Purcell is at your service.